THE INVISIBLE
ACHE

THE INVISIBLE ACHE

BLACK MEN IDENTIFYING THEIR PAIN AND RECLAIMING THEIR POWER

COURTNEY B. VANCE
and
DR. ROBIN L. SMITH
with **CHARISSE JONES**

balance

NEW YORK   BOSTON

Balance
Hachette Book Group
1290 Avenue of the Americas
New York, NY 10104
GCP-Balance.com
Twitter.com/GCPBalance
Instagram.com/GCPBalance

First Edition: November 2023

Balance is an imprint of Grand Central Publishing. The Balance name and logo are trademarks of Hachette Book Group, Inc.

The publisher is not responsible for websites (or their content) that are not owned by the publisher.

The Hachette Speakers Bureau provides a wide range of authors for speaking events. To find out more, go to hachettespeakersbureau.com or email HachetteSpeakers@hbgusa.com.

Balance books may be purchased in bulk for business, educational, or promotional use. For information, please contact your local bookseller or the Hachette Book Group Special Markets Department at special.markets@hbgusa.com.

Library of Congress Cataloging-in-Publication Data has been applied for.

ISBNs: 978-1-5387-2513-9 (hardcover), 978-1-5387-2515-3 (ebook)

Printed in the United States of America

LSC-C

Printing 1, 2023

*To my late father, Conroy Vance, and all the men who
have struggled in silence while doing their best to live
their lives out loud...let the light of your journeys be a
rainbow of hope for others seeking to find their way.*
—Courtney B. Vance

*To my late father, Warren E. Smith, MD, the first
man I loved who fiercely and without restraint loved
me in return—protected by his unapologetic and
uncompromising Black, brilliant, brave, and bold self,
body, mind, and spirit...paying and paving the way for
the fullest expression of the same DNA manifestation
in me. To Damian, my only brother, who, in layered
complexity, colored outside the lines in a world designed
to cage his soul's elegant Black body, brain, and burden.*
—Dr. Robin L. Smith

Contents

Introduction

While we need and seek solace in our bleakest moments, times of crisis can also push us to search for solutions. Along the way, the stars might fully align, bringing together a rare connection and partnership in which both individuals are driven by a similar and divine sense of urgency, compassion, and purpose. That's how this book came to be.

Courtney is no stranger to loss. When his father died by suicide, it shattered his heart and cracked his world open, launching him on his own mental health journey. Then, three decades later, it happened again. This time, it was his twenty-three-year-old godson who took his life. Courtney realized that he couldn't just look inward, working on himself in solitude. Black boys and men were suffering. Black boys and men were dying. He decided to share his personal struggles to show his brothers that there is no shame in hurting and no shame in healing, and that when you hurt or heal, you're not alone. No matter what you're going through, there are ways to regain your footing and create a life that is gratifying, honorable, and full.

Meanwhile, I have spent decades giving guidance to those navigating through trauma, or who are simply trying to be better partners, parents, and friends, all while riding life's myriad ups and downs. As I write these words, I consider how things have come full circle; my doctoral dissertation was entitled, "The Effects of Black Manhood Training on Adolescent African American Males." Throughout my career, I have been advocating for the inner and the outward empowerment of Black boys and girls long before it was fashionable. I've worked with youth and staff in the criminal justice system to further the health, wellness, and liberation of all parties trying to navigate systemic oppression and marginalization.

And yet what draws me to this work goes deeper than my professional training and practice. I am also a daughter, a sister, and a partner of Black men, and my learnings come, in part, from what I've witnessed and experienced living while Black within my family, in my skin, and the world.

When Courtney and I met a few years ago, we immediately began to talk about the alarming rise of suicides in the Black community. We lamented the firehose of negativity that comes at young people through social media. We shared righteous indignation over the effects of a once-in-a-century pandemic, a coarsely divided political culture, and a seemingly never-ending series of killings of Black men by police that were leaving so many anxious, depressed, hopeless, afraid, heartsick, and angry.

We ache for these men and their families. We ache for our society and our nation, which seem to be more lost with each day. We ache for ourselves, and our own families and communities around the diaspora who were very much impacted by chattel slavery, and which continues today.

The Invisible Ache is a first-step strategic response to the trauma that haunts so many Black boys and men, and those who love them and who are committed to their overall health and well-being. This book acts as a GPS, guiding Black boys and men toward better overall health and wholeness. Courtney and I see ourselves as first responders on the scene of crimes against the humanity and dignity of Black boys and men; *The Invisible Ache* offers a safe space to learn about and receive trauma-informed care, information, recovery, and renewal.

In these chapters, Courtney speaks first, mining his life, sharing his own traumas as well as his victories; his journey to prioritize self-care, his experiences in therapy and connecting with a psychologist who helped save his life and future. He speaks about how he learned to sit with loss and uncertainty, waiting for the mud to settle until the water became clear, and how he taught his children about the safe haven that therapy could be.

Building on Courtney's story, I offer guidance for how you can carve your own path to emotional wellness. You will learn vital questions to ask yourself to gain clarity about what may be hindering your confidence or the ability to attain your goals. You'll access resources you can tap when you are in distress, and ways you can be a safe sounding board for others, whether it's a friend, a family member, or a stranger you encounter during your day, who may be in need of help, guidance, or support.

Challenges are an integral part of life's journey, and to be mentally healthy is a lifelong quest. It is a goal that needs a renewed commitment each and every day. Yet achieving better emotional health is possible, especially when we share our pain and the tools that help us make it through.

Thankfully, in our modern era, the Black community is beginning to dismantle its historic stigma around mental illness and creating initiatives, networks, and organizations that are sources of support for Black men and boys who face an overwhelming onslaught of challenges, from the everyday pressures of school, work, and family, to microaggressions and overt acts of violence and hostility fueled by racism. Amid and despite it all, Black boys and men are reaching for and finding unmitigated joy, truth, and power, from the inside out.

Our hope is that this book becomes your companion, a touchstone and compass you turn to whenever you need it, to offer advice, to mirror your story, and most of all, to constantly remind you that you have a divine right to be fulfilled, happy, and whole. And in those moments when you know of others who may need the help and support, please share with them. Always remember that we are all in this together and that your full humanity is your complete and uncompromising divine and lawful birthright. You are worthy of all goodness, access, liberation, grace, and joy.

You are invited to come on this vital journey. Bring all of you—your wounds and your amazing survival narratives—and trust we will together reclaim for some, and claim anew for others, your power, your purpose, and your praise. As poet Derek Walcott wrote, you will come to "love again the stranger who was yourself."

There is a way to prevail from racism's vise grip. We will whisper what is true in safe and sacred spaces, and we will learn and relearn the foundational strategy and tool of telling your story, on the foundation of the West African proverb "The lion's story can never be known as long as the hunter is the one to tell it." Together, we will learn the necessity and value of Black boys and men knowing and telling their own story, never again having the hunter plagiarize and perpetuate a lie as the truth.

—Dr. Robin L. Smith

THE INVISIBLE ACHE

CHAPTER 1

Everybody's Got Issues

"Papa was like a shadow that was always hanging over me."

—CORY MAXSON, *FENCES*

It happened on a Wednesday.

I was costarring in *Six Degrees of Separation*, and the Vivian Beaumont Theater in Manhattan had been my second home for the last year and a half. I had a matinee that afternoon, another show to do in the evening, and a short break in between to catch my breath.

When the phone rang, I was lying in bed trying to shake off sleep and get my mind ready for my midweek hump. I fumbled for the receiver.

It was my mother calling. She was hysterical.

"Courtney!" she screamed. "It's your dad! He's dead!"

I leaped up.

"What?" I asked. "How?"

I was already reeling. But the words she said next nearly knocked me to my knees.

"He shot himself," she said, her screams lowering to a hush. "I found him. In the TV room."

There's no map for where your thoughts go in a moment like that, when you learn someone you can't imagine life without is now gone, not because he was snatched away by sickness or old age, but because he'd chosen to leave us, by his own hand.

My girlfriend, who'd been lying in bed beside me, sat up, stricken. How did she know? Could she hear my mother scream-ing? Had I somehow, in the seconds since the phone rang, sum-moned the strength to tell her the horrible news?

I can't recall. But I remember the next thought that ran through my mind. Call Stockard.

The wonderful actress Stockard Channing was playing Ouisa Kittredge, the Upper East Side socialite conned by my charac-ter, Paul, in *Six Degrees*. Given the intensity of our experiences doing that show, she was more than a costar. She'd become my comrade in arms.

To play Paul, a young man who insinuated himself into the posh lives of Kittredge and others in her world, I wanted the rhythm of my acting to mirror Paul's moves. I couldn't just memorize lines. I needed to scat, to play Paul fast and loose, performing the same way that he lived, improvising tall tales to entertain whoever was in front of him and making up a life as he went along.

Six Degrees had an unusual setup—cast members sat in the front row when they weren't onstage, allowing them to be a part of the audience. Inevitably, after every show, someone would bound toward me, slapping me on the back and shouting out praise for the great job I'd done. They had no idea that I was terrified by the thought I wasn't doing Paul justice and was con-stantly on the verge of walking out the side door and never com-ing back.

There were some performances where everything came

together. I was Paul. Paul was me. His deceptions and antics were as natural as if they'd been my own. Then there were nights where I felt the rhythm but not the words. I'd stand beneath the klieg lights, mouthing in rhythm nothing but gibberish until the words came back.

It took eight months for me to get to the point that I felt truly comfortable on that stage and was no longer clinging to a slippery slope. But once I got it, I was in the zone. It was like that for the other leads—Stockard and John Cunningham, who played Stockard's husband—as well. Our rhythm had been so hard to find, and our balance was so delicate to maintain, that we made a pact. We'd never take a day off. We'd never leave each other hanging. We'd take the stage together and harmonize every night.

Now my father was dead. I had to call Stockard.

I didn't have the mental strength to come up with a prelude, so I just blurted it out. "Stockard. My dad shot himself. He's dead."

Silence.

"Courtney," Stockard finally said. "Go home."

I could barely hear her. I was underwater.

"Courtney?...Courtney!" Stockard yelled. "Go home!"

I snapped out of my daze.

Slowly, my mind turned toward Northwest Detroit, the corner of the city where my parents bought their first house. I began to think about how I needed to get home, to plan a funeral, to take care of my mother.

My girlfriend and I had been together for roughly a decade at that point, studying drama at Yale, then taking our first steps into life as professional actors on the regional stages all over the country, before making it to Manhattan. She'd been my anchor, encouraging and protecting me. I'd never forgotten how she had words with our fellow acting students at Yale when many became resentful of my early success.

So, on the most devastating day of my life, it was she, of course, who got me together. She rubbed my shoulders and took me in her arms, mustering every ounce of energy she could to keep me from crashing and unmooring even more.

I don't remember the in between, but somehow, we booked a flight for me and I got to LaGuardia Airport. When the taxi pulled up to 15096 Appoline Street, the house where I'd hung Christmas stockings and practiced free throws in the driveway looked unfamiliar. I gazed at the front door, not wanting to imagine what I'd find on the other side.

I was thirty years old, but I felt like a boy suddenly dealing with big man stuff. And the big man I would typically turn to for advice had taken his own life.

Death had come to me just once before, when I was sixteen, when a friend of mine was killed. I can't remember how he died, only how those who knew him mourned. The musk of roses, the drone of prayers, the quiet sobbing in the back of the packed church. It was the only funeral I'd ever been to.

It was unbelievable that a boy I'd shared jokes with and sat beside in class was now lying in front of me in a casket. When the service was over, I pushed that image way back in my memory. I didn't have time to waste worrying and reflecting. I had to keep moving forward, I had to keep on achieving, just like my mother and father had taught me to.

For thirty years, I'd been able to avoid the vicissitudes of life, putting all my energy into excelling at school and in my career. From the campus of Country Day, the prestigious prep school in Michigan I started attending in the ninth grade, to the Ivy-shadowed halls of Harvard and Yale, to the cramped, gilded theaters of Broadway, I felt I'd done all that I was supposed to.

It was my sister, Cecilie, who'd struggled as a teenager, battling bouts of depression, even occasionally running away from home before the realization of how harsh life on the streets would be drove her back to our parents' arms. She'd been the fragile one in the family. Dad, charismatic and wise, was always the voice of calm, the ballast holding us steady.

Yet somehow Dad had been the one to break. The psychologist who would eventually give me counsel, who would help me learn myself and teach me how to sit in silence and wait for the water to clear, gave me the frame through which I could begin to understand the devastating choice he'd made.

It was during a session when, between the notes of sadness, I'd also remembered moments of joy. I told the psychologist how blessed I'd been to be able to act with legends and luminaries like Mary Alice and James Earl Jones.

My therapist looked at me.

"But I'll bet you never knew that your father was actually the greatest actor you'd ever met," she said.

I didn't respond. I had nothing to say.

––––––––

I loved my father deeply, but I hardly knew him.

My mother, Leslie, was a Daniels and I took after that side of the family with my round nose and wide eyes. Daddy, sturdy and a few inches shy of six feet, had an angular nose and sharp cheekbones, like a copper-hued Greek statue.

From architecture to politics, there wasn't a subject Conroy Vance couldn't talk about. He filled any room he walked into, enchanting you with a smile or a joke, leaving you dizzy as you tried to keep up with his maze of thought. He and my sister would banter back and forth about whatever Walter Cronkite was discussing on the evening news or the front-page headlines in the *Detroit Free Press*. But I would hold back, too intimidated by Dad's intellect to ever debate him. I wouldn't even play chess with him because, though I wanted to learn, I didn't want to get my behind kicked into oblivion whenever I pulled a chair up to the board.

I'm sure he wanted me to engage, to express myself, but I was afraid to take him on, not because he was condescending or mean but because he seemed invincible. I just wanted to watch, to listen, and to bask in his brilliance.

But there was a time when I did speak up. It is one of my most enduring memories.

I was in high school and my cousin Evie and I were riding back from some errand in Dad's big sunshine yellow van. The CB radio he loved was crackling, and in between the cryptic jargon that only he and his CB brothers and sisters could understand, Dad asked me a question. Would I go fight in Vietnam?

In 1974, Saigon had yet to fall, and so a war that began five years before I was born was still roaring when I was in high school. More than 58,000 Americans would ultimately lose their lives there, a disproportionate number of them poor and Black.

Typically, I would have mumbled, "I don't know," or "I don't really want to talk about it," and hoped Dad would shrug and turn his attention back to his radio. But something welled up inside me that day. I wanted to discuss it; I wanted to debate.

Hell no, I didn't want to go to Vietnam.

"I won't fight," I said, finding my voice. "I'm going to college. I'm not risking my life for a war ten thousand miles away."

It was on.

"You are an American," he said. "This is about fighting communism and defending democracy. You don't want to do that?"

"All I know is I don't want to lose my life before it's even really started," I snapped back. "I want to have time to discover what I want to do. That can't happen if I'm over in Vietnam, dead."

We pulled up in front of our house, still battling. Evie, sitting in the back seat, said she had to go and hopped out. Soon my mother was knocking on the window, looking at us like we had lost our minds.

"What are you doing?" she asked.

"We're talking," Dad and I said in unison.

"Well," she said, shaking her head, "come talk in the house."

It went on like that for hours, Dad and I jousting and jabbing. We'd finished dinner and the dishes were drying by the sink when Dad and I sat slouched against cushions in the living room, continuing our dissection of foreign policy as we struggled to keep our eyes open. Finally, Mommy had had enough.

"Conroy," she said, exasperated. "The war will still be going on tomorrow. Let the boy go to bed."

Reluctantly, Dad and I rose from the couch. We each had one more thing to say.

"I love you, Daddy," I said before heading upstairs to my room.

"I love you too, Son," he said, a smile creasing his tired face.

That love, his love, was never in doubt. My sister and I were loved beyond measure, rocked to sleep by it, steeped in it. Our father, however, hadn't grown up with such comfort.

There was a picture tucked in the back of one of our family albums. It was a photo of my dad taken when he was a little boy living in the foster home where he spent his earliest years. The other children were all pale, probably the offspring of white mothers and Black fathers, dropped off and discarded to keep them hidden from sight. Daddy was the only brown-skinned one in the bunch, part of the group but also apart from it, different and alone.

I was married with two children of my own when I began to unravel the story of my father's beginnings. My wife, the incredible actress Angela Bassett, and I sat down with the scholar Henry Louis Gates for an episode of his series *Finding Your Roots*. On the show, Gates unearthed the ancestry of his guests, and for years, actors, musicians, and other celebrities had been discovering the Civil War soldiers, suffragettes, and stowaways who'd been their elders.

When it was my turn, I learned about a girl named Ardella.

When Ardella was fifteen, she delivered a baby boy. At the time, birth certificates noted how many stillbirths the mother had had previously. Ardella's baby's certificate said his mother had had six. Six stillbirths. At fifteen. So somebody was messing with that child, raping her, from the time she was nine years old.

This baby boy thankfully would live. She named him Larry. But Ardella, a little Black girl molested since she was in knee socks, a child who'd delivered dead baby after dead baby, had a mind that was all messed up. So they took Larry, her first child to survive, and gave him to her sister to raise. Larry didn't find out until he was nineteen years old that his mama was really his aunt.

Then, a year or two later, Ardella had another son, Conroy. But there was nobody in the family who could raise him, so he was put in foster care. He eventually was taken in by a couple and found some semblance of a home, but my daddy lived his whole life thinking that his real mama didn't want him.

When our episode of *Finding Your Roots* aired, relatives on my father's side reached out to myself and my sister. During our reunion, we heard stories about how the family sent Ardella to Arkansas to live for a while. When she returned to Chicago, she was older, but time away hadn't healed her mind. She'd walk around the house talking to herself.

"They took my Conroy," she'd murmur. "They took my Conroy."

She was missing her boy. She'd loved him. She'd wanted him. She wanted to know, Where is the boy you took from me? She never would find out.

Ardella and my father were tormented by each other's absence. My mother told me once how Daddy got a faraway look in his eyes one afternoon when they were driving through Chicago.

"I know this street," he said, gazing out the window.

"What is it, Conroy?" she asked him. "What's on your mind?" But he wouldn't tell her. He kept the haunting to himself, and he carried all that hurt to an early grave.

My daddy ended his life thinking his mama gave him up, that she threw him away. If my father could have just gotten the support he needed to help him hold on a little longer, he would have been reunited with his family. He could have met his brother Larry and his grandchildren who had yet to be born. He would have discovered that his Chicago family had been looking for him all this time, and how happy Ardella, now dead, would have been to know that they'd finally found her boy.

That's why it's not our call to take ourselves out. You just don't know what God has in store for you. But to hold on, you have to learn how to befriend and quiet the ghosts. You need the tools so you can tunnel through the pain, make it out the other side, and thrive.

———

Though *Six Degrees* was an indelible part of my theater career, I'd made my Broadway debut in *Fences*, the August Wilson play that went on to win a Pulitzer Prize, a bunch of Tony Awards, and got me my first Tony nomination. I was Cory Maxson, the son of a sanitation worker played by James Earl Jones, and Mary Alice was my mother, Rose.

"Papa was a shadow that was always hanging over me," my character, Cory, said on stage, night after night.

Rose would then put her hand on my shoulder. "That shadow wasn't nothing but you, growing into yourself," she said. "You've got to take the best of what's in a person and the rest of it you've got to let go. You've got to take the best of what was in him and go on with your life."

It was not the last time my art would mirror my reality. And I would eventually understand that I had to do like Rose said, taking her wisdom to heart.

From the time I was thirteen years old, I was away from home sixteen hours a day. That was the sacrifice for going to Country Day, the prestigious school that transformed my life.

I was getting a first-class education that would pave my path to two of the most highly regarded colleges in the world and enable me to form relationships with students who would grow up to be titans of business and sports. But it meant that when I was home, there was just enough time left to eat, do some homework, and get a few hours of sleep. I was busy achieving, which was what my parents raised me to do. They wanted me to be honored, to be lifted, to do all the things that they, my mother working as a librarian, and my father, a Chrysler benefits administrator, couldn't.

Like so many of my peers, I was carrying the dreams of all the Black folks who'd endured so much, fighting for respect and just an inkling of an opportunity. Just as I knew to brush my teeth when I woke up in the morning and to say my prayers before I went to bed, I understood that I would need to study and excel in whatever I did. That was how my generation, children handed the torch from parents and grandparents who fled the violence and indignities of the South, were raised.

Work hard, our elders told us. Stay focused. Be disciplined. What are you looking at the floor for? There's nothing down there. Aim for the sky.

Still, for a long time, I sensed my father was in crisis. though I didn't know what to do with the knowing.

Daddy kept his hurt to himself. Neither he nor my mother were ones to gripe or complain in front of their children. But there was an unease in the air, hovering in between all the words left unsaid. I would come home from school and Daddy would be downstairs in his office while Mom was upstairs in their bedroom. I would go back and forth between the two of them, trying to be a bridge, trying to mend something I didn't understand but that I felt was broken all the same.

I think my dad wanted to be an attorney when he was young, but his foster father spent my dad's tuition money. Dad had to go into the Air Force and rely on the G.I. Bill to help him pay for school. As smart as he was, he was often bored in class and his high school grades were lackluster. I wondered sometimes if he would have tried harder and earned a scholarship if he'd known that the money he assumed would be there for college had been squandered on his foster dad's new car, a vacation or two or three, and other trivial things that wouldn't last, and didn't matter.

However deep that wound, or maybe because of it, Dad determined that it would be different for me. When I went through his things after he died, I learned that his credit cards were maxed out, not a dollar left among them.

But he'd paid off one debt. It was the loan he and my mother took out to pay my way through Harvard.

———

My grandfather spent my dad's tuition money and didn't leave him anything but bills. But there was one inheritance. Guns. A whole lot of guns.

My mother would complain, saying she couldn't understand why Dad kept all those damn rifles and pistols. They sat on a shelf in a closet nestled among baseball caps, Christmas decorations, and empty shoeboxes. There wasn't a need for them. We lived in a safe neighborhood and Daddy didn't hunt. But he wouldn't get rid of them. After he killed himself, I understood why.

I now believe that the thought of suicide was planted in my father's mind as soon as he was old enough to know it was a possibility because he was so scarred by his mother's absence. And when the idea of taking your life becomes an option, it never leaves you unless you replace that mental loop with something as positive as those life ending thoughts are bleak.

The mind is so fragile. Some people take their pain out on others. Some inflict it all on themselves. Feeling as much pain as he endured in his life, as much loss and longing, it's a miracle Dad lasted as long as he did. Still, I don't think there was any one of us, in our family, among my father's circle of friends, who ever imagined he would take things so far.

When I got the call that my father was dead and I flew home, I found my mother puddled up on the floor. It took a couple days for my sister to get to Michigan, so I nursed Mom's grief and my own mostly alone. In the coming days, Mommy somehow gathered herself enough to call the funeral director, and during the homegoing ceremony she nodded her head through the hymns and eulogies and picked at her plate during the repast.

After the service was over, I wanted to run back to my life. School had been a gift from my parents, a responsibility I had to fulfill, but it was also my escape, a way to avoid whatever was going on in our home. Now, as I performed on Broadway, my career filled the same void. I wanted to get back to work and push the picture of my father's casket so deep in my subconscious that I could hardly find it. I was ready to roar through, to rise higher, like I'd always done. Like my parents taught me to.

But where there had been four, there were now just us three. And my mother was ready to teach me something different.

I'd just finished packing my bag for New York when Mom called my sister and me into the living room and asked us to sit down.

"When you both get back home, I want each of you to go to therapy," she said. "And I'm going to find me someone to talk with too."

She didn't want us to keep the pain a secret, not our father's, not our own.

You don't want to wait until a tragedy happens to realize you've got stuff to get over. It took my father killing himself for me to recognize I had issues. We all do. And we've all got to figure out what those issues are, and face them. If we don't, they will overtake us, stamp out our light, and leave a trail of broken hearts behind. One of those broken hearts will probably be your own.

My old way of coping, the escaping, the not dealing with, the rising above, had gotten me to the age of thirty. But after my mother found my father's limp body, I learned the old ways had taken me as far as they could. I had to do something different.

I never realized I needed therapy. I didn't even really know what therapy was. But my mother asked me to get some. And I always did what my mother and father told me.

"Okay, Mommy," I said. "I'll get some help."

But how to begin?

An Invitation

When I met Courtney, it had been thirty years since his father's suicide. Still, I intuitively understood his story, and that of his father.

Their stories echoed the pressures of so many Black men I'd known who were dealing with feelings of abandonment and shame, depression and grief, and the aftermath of secrets and suicide.

For Black men, such emotions and experiences are compounded by the brutal reality of racism. Going up against such forces is like trying to stay on your feet in the face of a gale wind, and all those stresses are taking a tremendous toll on Black men's mental health. Yet too many suffer alone.

When there are discussions about mental well-being, at conferences, at retreats, or during late-night seminars that air on public TV, the faces are typically white, and if there's someone of color in the mix, that person is usually female. But Courtney and I want to change that. We are issuing an invitation to Black men to join the conversation because they need and deserve to be at the table.

There are cultural barriers that have prevented both Black men and women from voicing their inner turmoil. When you feel pressured every day to refute the lies that you are lazy or incompetent, you also feel pressured to live up to the belief that Black people are preternaturally strong physically and mentally. Indeed, that's a stereotype we may even take pride in. The resilience it has taken to survive in a nation that literally once regarded us as animals, breaking our bodies for capital, stealing our children, and brutalizing us for sport, is indeed remarkable and worthy of praise.

There is also a particular fortitude and grace required to walk through the world as a Black man. You are targeted and burdened in a way that is especially ugly and unique. For white men, their race along with their gender grants them protection as well as privilege. But Black men are literally hounded and hunted—physically, mentally, and emotionally—every day because of who they are.

When you have been portrayed as dangerous and lacking, you learn to live life on defense. You glower and bluster, using hypermasculinity like a shield. Whether you are a corporate lawyer holding sway in a boardroom, or a teenage boy hanging out on a street corner, posturing becomes a life preserver. And many men feel talking about how they hurt would shatter their carefully constructed masks, leaving them even more vulnerable.

That's why until recently it's been relatively rare for a famous, successful Black man like Courtney to bare their pain in public, to admit that despite all the peaks in their life and career, they've been mired in emotional valleys too. It may be harder still for the working-class boy on the playground, the brother trying to get on his feet after a stint in jail, or the student making the grades in an all-white world to acknowledge their own emotional fragility.

But struggle and doubt are sections in the braid of life, as integral to our corporeal existence as love, passion, and those precious moments of unadulterated joy. Our broken parts when pieced together are what make us human and whole. The emotional burdens that break us down are also the same obstacles that can teach the lessons and grant the perspective that allow us after the gale wind wanes and we've survived the storm, to stand tall, look out, and marvel at how we got over insurmountable obstacles.

THE OTHER PANDEMIC

COVID-19 shut the world down, but there is another pandemic that merits urgent attention—the mental health crisis leading to rising rates of depression and anxiety among Black boys and men.

Major depressive episodes with severe impairment among young Black men between the ages of 18 and 25 rose from 2.5% in 2015 to 4.3% in 2018, according to the 2018 National Survey on Drug Use and Health by the Substance Abuse and Mental Health Services Administration.*

Suicide and suicidal ideation, the thought of not being here or yearning for it all to be over, are also becoming more prevalent. According to the Centers for Disease Control and Prevention's Youth Risk Behavior Survey published in 2019, Black students between the ages of 14 and 18 represented 11.8% of the youths in that group who said they'd attempted to take their own lives. Meanwhile, their white peers comprised 7.9% of that cohort, and Hispanic teens represented 8.9% of those who said they'd attempted suicide.

---

* 2018 National Survey on Drug Use and Health: African Americans. Substance Abuse and Mental Health Services Administration, U.S. Department of Health and Human Services, Jan. 14, 2020. https://www.samhsa.gov/data /sites/default/files/reports/rpt23247/2_AfricanAmerican_2020_01_14_508 .pdf.

More broadly, while suicide rates for non-Hispanic whites were two to three times greater than for non-Hispanic Black people from 2000 through 2020, the trajectory has begun to shift. Age-adjusted suicide rates among non-Hispanic Black people dropped from 5.6% in 2000 to 5.1% in 2007, but then rose to 7.8% in 2020—a 53% increase. Meanwhile, age-adjusted suicide rates among non-Hispanic whites, which rose 51% between 2000 and 2018, dropped 7% from 2018 through 2020.[*]

In 2021, the suicide rate among Black people rose again, to 8.7%, a 19.2% spike as compared to the previous year, according to the Centers for Disease Control and Prevention. The surging suicide rate—from 8.2% to 11.2%—among Black Americans between the ages of 10 and 24 from 2018 through 2021 caused the CDC particular concern.[†] Yet as alarming as these numbers are, the reality is likely even worse. There continues to be a need for more research on the causes and ramifications of Black trauma. And so, just as we can be sure that the number of Africans who were kidnapped and brought to this part of the world was far higher than the 12 million people historians claim, we can be certain that the number of Black men who are

---

[*] Sally C. Curtin, Kamiah A. Brown, and Mariah E. Jordan, "Suicide Rates for the Three Leading Methods by Race and Ethnicity: 2000–2020." NCHS Data Brief No. 450, National Center for Health Statistics, CDC, Nov. 2022. https://www.cdc.gov/nchs/products/databriefs/db450.htm.

[†] Deborah M. Stone, Karin A. Mack, and Judith Qualters, "Notes from the Field: Recent Changes in Suicide Rates, by Race and Ethnicity and Age Group—United States, 2021." *Morbidity and Mortality Weekly Report*, CDC, Feb. 10, 2023. https://www.cdc.gov/mmwr/volumes/72/wr/mm7206a4.htm?s_cid=mm7206a4_w.

struggling and in need of support is far greater than what has been recorded.

Whatever statistics we include in this book reflect only the people who showed up for the study, who were counted in the sample, who were open enough to their emotions to acknowledge their pain to a stranger.

Among Black Americans, just one in three who need mental health support actually get it, according to a 2017 fact sheet from the American Psychiatric Association. And for Black men, candor and reaching out for help can be especially difficult.

It is hard, because Black men are consumed by a definition of themselves imposed by others. As Isabel Wilkerson noted in her seminal book, *Caste*, they are constrained by an American racial hierarchy that has become a literal tomb, etching them in stereotype and denying them their full humanity.

The idea that Black men are violent and unworthy is cruel and untrue, yet it has the power to swallow a man whole, becoming the operating system for how the world treats him, and sometimes, tragically, dictating how he sees and treats himself.

Those lies are the fuel for the machinery that funnels Black boys into a criminal justice system that literally profits from their confinement and debasement, an apparatus that starts churning in the guidance counseling offices and crowded halls of elementary schools before delivering them to crippling sentences in juvenile detention centers and state prisons.

Constantly being eyed with suspicion and derision leaves many anxious, tense, and resentful. But Black men's trauma can play hide and seek. Maybe your nephew doesn't make an overt attempt to take his own life, but he smokes a blunt first thing in the morning, or drinks Hennessy until he collapses, his body slack and his mind numb. Perhaps he overindulges in food, or sex or work. Or maybe he barely works at all, not wanting to engage with a hostile world, content to let someone else carry the burden since he feels he already has enough crosses to bear. Maybe this is you.

Whichever path he takes, they are all ways to build a buffer between his feelings and the wounding he so often endures. They are ways to take cover against the onslaught. And whether he means to or not, he is killing himself slowly.

NO ONE SHOULD HAVE TO BE SUPERMAN

Black women deal with many similar pressures, from the dehumanizing assumption they are too tough to need comfort, to mistreatment at the hands of an often racist health care system that overlooks their physical as well as mental pain.

As the mothers, lovers, and daughters of Black men, Black women have been their biggest allies, walking beside them, lifting them up. But at times they can be excessively critical too, their barbs stemming from the frustration they feel when their expectations of what a man is supposed to be, as defined by a racist, misogynistic society, aren't fully met.

"He doesn't get me and what I'm needing."

"He doesn't tell me how he feels."

"I'm trying to make this work, but he just doesn't show up."

It's completely normal to express frustration with your partner, but Black men are so accustomed to having people disappointed in them that when their sisters are dismissive, they often put up even more of a wall. When Black women lash out or withdraw, their partners, fathers, and brothers have yet another reason to shut down. They may separate even more from their emotions, and the detachment that was criticized in the first place becomes a self-fulfilling prophecy.

And then there's the flip side of disappointment and criticism, which can be just as stifling.

I recall speaking to the wife of one of the many Black men who are out there shepherding their children, making a good living, and creating a legacy. She beamed with pride that her husband had it all together. She marveled at how he and so many others like him didn't let society's prejudices and judgments beat him down, how he'd figured out how to manage and succeed in a hostile world. But she never asked what that cost him, not because she didn't care, but because she didn't realize that his aura of infallibility was a mask that he didn't take off, even with her.

As a friend, a sister, a daughter, a therapist, and ordained clergy, I, too, see how hard Black men are working. I also bear witness to how exhausted many of them are. I think about what it means for them to be assaulted, not just physically like Tyre Nichols, George Floyd, Trayvon Martin, and all the others that went before and who will, infuriatingly, come after, but what it means to face and navigate psychological violence every day—when you try to hail a cab that won't stop, encounter a store clerk who treats you like a thief, or pass a white woman who shifts her purse to the other side of her body when you walk by.

What is the toll of maintaining your decorum amid such microaggressions? What is the mental cost of trying to forget about that daily tightrope so you don't lash out at the world or collapse within yourself and combust?

So many Black men feel reckoning with that emotional jiujitsu would sacrifice their sanity. But denial is yet another burden, robbing us of the mental and emotional energy that we could use to create, to imagine, and to seek out what brings us happiness.

SILENCE ISN'T GOLDEN

Shame has a unique manifestation in Black men, who must constantly fight to be fully seen as the complete beings that they are. Many feel that to articulate those delicate parts of themselves, their tenderness, and their faults, is a sign of weakness. They don't shine a light on their jagged, imperfect pieces in order to protect themselves from harm and derision.

Even Black men who have triumphed in the conventional ways that success is measured, often carry the burden of making sure they don't slip. That they don't take a step, make a move, or utter a word that allows a hostile world to pass judgment. They are terrified of succumbing to a false definition made up by someone who wants them to fail and suffer.

But contrary to the old adage, silence isn't golden. It is actually deadly. So let's talk it out.

Black men should feel free to talk to each other about their emotional struggles, to shatter the stigma around mental illness and to let each other know that they are not alone. Black men can learn a new language that allows them to articulate the roots of their pain, and to narrate their journey toward wellness, because there is no one-stop cure. There is no miracle that will suddenly make them whole. They must intentionally, consciously tend to their emotional wounds every day. Healing is a spiritual journey that begins the moment you realize what you are trying to work through, and it will continue until you take your last breath.

It's not easy to probe so deep. It's certainly not been easy to seek quality care from a health care system riven with discrimination and injustice, from the theft of Henrietta Lacks's cells to the infamous Tuskegee Experiment. You don't even have to go back in history to see those disparities play out. Still too often, the emotional and physical pain of Black people is ignored or denied.

Yes, the health care system needs to root out bias and offer more accessible, culturally relevant care. Yes, the government and broader society needs to remedy inequities to repay those who were so critical to the building of this nation and strengthen our society as a whole. But Black people are not sitting idly by, putting their healing on hold. We are increasingly realizing that we are the ones we have been waiting for. And as our ancestors proclaimed, each one can teach and reach one.

Courtney has a right not to share his story. But if he were to say his father died, and not tell you how, if he were to say he needed help but not the steps he took to get it, his story would be only half told. And he would not be living in, and growing from, his truth, or helping others to find theirs.

Wholeness, in the way many of us think of it, is a myth. To be whole is not to be perfect. Courtney, like me, like all of us, still has plenty of cracks in need of filling. But what Courtney has discovered, what he and I hope every Black boy and man we touch will realize as well, is that wholeness is really about showing up, not just for others but, most importantly, for yourself.

CHAPTER 2

Where Does It Hurt?

"Do you have the patience to wait till your mud settles and the water is clear? Can you remain unmoving till the right action arises by itself?"

—LAO TZU

I had no clue how to find a therapist. Did you pick up the phone book, close your eyes, and call whatever name your finger landed on? Would the ideal doctor pop up in a commercial one night when I was up late watching TV?

When I was away at Harvard, my sister began seeing a psychologist, whom I believe she was referred to by a high school counselor. But as far as I knew, no one else in my life had ever gone to therapy. I figured that Cecilie had been an exception to the unspoken rule that you just persevered and carried on, exemplified by my parents' dedication to work and family, and reinforced by all those civil rights documentaries we watched growing up that showed Black folks being brave and steady.

Finally, because I had no idea how else to do it, I wound up simply asking friends and colleagues if they could recommend someone. I was surprised by how many had suggestions. I also quickly found out that getting someone's name and booking an appointment was going to be the easiest part of my search.

The first therapist I went to see was a Black woman with a soothing voice, who purred from her perch in a wide brown chair. Pen and notebook in hand, she sat across from me as I squeezed into the corner of a small couch. Then, for most of the next hour, we just sat there looking at each other.

At one point, I leaned over and held my head in my hands.

"Do you have a headache?" she asked.

Was she serious? I looked up, exasperated. "No, I don't have a headache," I said through clenched teeth. "I don't know how to do this therapy thing, and you're not helping me. How do I do this?"

I guess that stumped her because she went silent. Our staring contest continued until our session mercifully came to an end.

One thing I knew for sure—she wasn't the therapist for me. But now I had to keep looking, and I felt overwhelmed trying to find the right someone when I wasn't entirely sure what I was looking for.

I made appointments with a few other doctors. There was the amiable guy in the plaid jacket who seemed more interested in my diet and exercise routine than he was in getting to the roots of my grief. Then there was the redhead who might as well have had a timer on her desk, given how she told me we had exactly one hour and kept checking the clock, determined not to give me one minute more.

I was still performing in *Six Degrees*, and my castmates provided a cocoon where I could briefly forget my pain. I didn't want to talk to any of them about my dad's suicide. I didn't know what to say. But I began getting massages every Wednesday in between the matinee and the evening show to try to calm my frazzled nerves.

Laura Linney was one of my colleagues. She's a superstar now, of course, with credits stretching from *Ozark* to *Frasier*, but back in 1990, she was an understudy ready to take the lead if Stockard or other *Six Degrees* cast members were unable to perform. She knew about my Wednesday routine, and one day she told me that she had a great masseuse I should try.

Her name was Gunilla Asp, and Laura's recommendation turned out to be one of the greatest gifts anyone has ever given me.

When I got to Gunilla's studio, she left me alone to undress and settle myself on the massage table. I was nestling my face into the head rest when she reentered the room.

"Before we start," she said. "Is there anything I should know?"

It was the routine question all massage therapists asked. You were supposed to tell them about the tender tendon in your calf, the old sports injury that wrecked your shoulder, or the ache in your lower back that came from sitting behind a desk all day.

I told Miss Gunilla about the ache in my heart instead.

"Well," I said. "My daddy died of suicide about a month ago."

Then I broke down.

Gunilla pulled me up and hugged me, her tears mixing with mine. Then, she gently told me to lie back down. She soothed my tired muscles with oil, pressed her thumbs into my joints until the tension drained away, and finally rocked me to the brink of sleep.

When our session was over and I emerged from the room, she offered me a cup of tea and a piece of paper with a name.

"I know a therapist who I think would be perfect for you," she said.

Her name was Margaret Kornfeld. I was beginning to doubt there was any therapist who was right for me, let alone perfect. But Miss Gunilla and I had been so in tune, I tried to muster a bit of hope. I called Dr. Kornfeld's office and scheduled an appointment for the following Monday, my one day off from the play.

The night before I met Dr. K, I had a dream. I seldom remembered what went through my mind as I slept. Sometimes there would be bits and pieces that stayed in my consciousness the following day and I'd stop for a moment wondering if I was experiencing an actual memory or just recalling a sliver of a slumber-fueled fairy tale. But that Monday, an image stayed with me. I'd seen a pillow decorated with an unusual pattern.

I took a cab over to the Gramercy Park area of Manhattan and walked the two floors up to Dr. K's office. There was a room to the right that was a bit sterile with a desk and chair, and then a room to the left with a couch.

A pillow was propped against the larger cushions. It was decorated with the same spidery pattern I'd seen in my dream.

I was dumbstruck. It had to be a sign. This was where I was meant to be.

"Hello," a petite, brown-haired Jewish woman suddenly said, extending her hand. "I'm Dr. Kornfeld."

"The pillow! On the couch," I said, my sentences running together. "The pattern on it. I saw that last night! In a dream!"

I followed her into the room with the couch, rambling a mile a minute. My father killed himself, I explained. My mother told me to get counseling. I've never done this before. I didn't know how to feel.

When I finally stopped long enough to take a sip of water, Dr. K spoke her first words since our greeting.

"Courtney," she said softly. "You don't have to tell me everything today."

"Okay," I said, still excited but now also a little embarrassed. "I just need to talk."

I needed to talk even though I didn't know what about. I needed to talk to someone who would listen and help me unpack the layers. I needed someone who could help decipher the clues. I'd needed to talk for thirty years. And before that day, I'd never known there was a woman like Dr. K who was even an option for me to talk to.

———

During my junior year at Harvard, the actress Cathy Slade suggested I try out for a theater troupe called Shakespeare & Company. That summer, after I'd been accepted, I headed to a farm in Massachusetts where I and fifteen other apprentices would spend six weeks together working on our craft.

I was still testing out the stage, trying to figure out if this was a hobby or something I might want to stick with as a career, so my understanding of acting was rudimentary. I thought it was basically mimicking accents and emotions and I was getting pretty good.

But Tina Packer, artistic director of Shakespeare & Company, expected much more. During our second or third day there, she walked to the front of the room.

"Now people," she said to quiet our nervous chatter. "I would like each of you to come up here and one at a time tell the group two things you want us to know about yourself."

Hmmm, I thought. Maybe I'll mention how much I enjoy sports. Or how I love nothing more than to get up before dawn so I can sit in silence and just listen to the birds.

Miss Packer wasn't finished.

"And," she said, pausing dramatically, "I want you to tell us two things you don't want us to know about yourself."

Everyone in the room froze.

"What does she want us to do?" I thought.

My mind went into a tailspin. Why on earth would I tell a bunch of folks I barely knew some deep, dark secret? I hurriedly tried to come up with something I could say that seemed private but that I really didn't mind sharing. It was the first of many unsettling moments my fellow apprentices and I would have that summer. Ms. Packer and the other faculty challenged us to come so far out of our comfort zones that, at times, I was hanging mentally by a thread. She forced me to go into emotional crevices where I didn't want to go, to think about my fears, to challenge my insecurities.

I began to question acting. What was this thing that had chosen me? Being on the stage felt so natural in the beginning but now I was no longer sure I wanted to see it through.

One night I darted out of my room. We were so deep in the woods that you had to walk half a mile to get to a road. I was scared of the dark, but I was more afraid of the emotional path acting was beginning to take me on. I had to get out. I felt like running. I found my way to the road, walked a mile, grabbed a stop sign pole, shook it, and screamed.

But that's what great acting was really about. It didn't take a lot to imitate a voice, to put on a costume, or to memorize a script. If you wanted to truly connect with folks in the audience, to make them believe, you had to believe it too. You had to feel, to go to that place inside yourself that was fragile and soft and human.

It hurt. It was uncomfortable. And eventually that inner

journey would prove to be clarifying, not only on the stage but, most importantly, in my real, everyday life.

————————

I'd been seeing Dr. K for about a month when she asked me a question.

"Courtney," she said in her gentle voice. "How do you make decisions?"

I'd never really thought about it. In the theater I'd developed the ability to tap into my emotions at will. So I figured that was how I ticked offstage as well.

"I guess I just leap in, like when I'm acting," I said. "I just flip a coin and go for it. That's the way most people do it, right?"

Dr. K understood there had to be a lot more to my decision making than that. Did I really want to be a jumper who leapt into the abyss, hoping there was somebody down there to catch me? Or did I want to have the patience to sit down and let the solution rise up within me in its own time?

"Flipping a coin or leaping feet first may be great for acting, but do you think that really works when you're dealing with difficult situations in your life?" she asked.

Dr. K then quoted a sage named Lao Tzu, someone I'd never heard of but whose wisdom I can no longer live without.

"Do you have the patience to let the mud settle in the water and the water become clear?" she said.

What Lao Tzu and Dr. K understood is that sometimes you can't do anything. Sometimes your mind is cloudy or your compass is out of whack. You have to prepare for those situations where you can only just sit and wait for the answer, for the clarity and peace to come, however long it takes. Because if you jump, your world will fracture. Maybe you'll even die.

She wanted me to drill down and understand how I processed both the routine and the challenging experiences that would inevitably come my way. Maybe if I'd been able to hang in an uncomfortable place for a minute and wait for the water to become clear, my relationship with my longtime girlfriend would have had a less turbulent ending. Who knew? It was a mystery. In many ways, I was a mystery. But I loved my sessions with Dr. K, where I began to tackle the riddle that was my self.

"This here is my time," I'd think as I settled in every Monday, leaning against that pillow that was the first clue I was in the right place. "I can talk about anything I want to."

When I was at Country Day, I was an all-around athlete, playing football, basketball, and running track, high hurdles, and long jump. I was up early, running laps, and spent my afternoons practicing drills, shooting free throws, and working on whatever, depending on the season. Like so many athletes, I reveled in working out and working hard, partly because the reward was so visceral. When you do the work physically, you're a superstar. You're admired for being svelte and strong. After the game or the meet, you're treated like a gladiator returning victoriously from war. The payoff is immediate.

So many of us are willing to work out physically, or to put long hours and effort into our professional careers. We work on everything but our mental and emotional health. But if those two areas aren't right, you can be the biggest superstar in the world, the finest specimen walking, and still be in the midst of hell.

The stage was my safe space because I knew what to do there. But when the performing was done, I still had to live, and that was harder than doing two shows a day, engaging in all-night rehearsals, or reciting the most tongue-twisting monologue Shakespeare ever wrote.

Dr. K was helping me to excavate my emotions not for an audience, but for myself. She was teaching me to write my own script and not merely recite somebody else's. I had to find a safe space that wasn't rooted in make-believe. I had to know and be comfortable within myself, wherever I was. I want my Black brothers, each and every one of them, to find that peace as well.

In our fourth or fifth meeting, Dr. K returned to where our journey began.

"Tell me about your dreams," she said.

"I told you about the pattern on the pillow," I said, a little startled. "But that was unusual. I don't really remember anything when I wake up in the morning."

She paused.

"Well," she said, with a slight smile. "I need you to go catch your dreams."

A Vital Tool

I started practicing psychology more than thirty years ago, and through the decades I've worked with hundreds of patients dealing with a myriad of challenges, from troubled relationships to instances of abuse. As a Black woman who's been both a clinician and a patient, I've also encountered many myths.

"Therapy is for white folks."

"Black people don't need no psychiatrist."

"Take your worries to God. Prayer is enough."

Perhaps because gender stereotypes give women a little more latitude to express their need for emotional support, Black women were initially more willing to publicly share the healing they've experienced through counseling. More recently, however, celebrated Black men like Courtney and *Black Panther* star Michael B. Jordan have also recounted their journeys with therapy. In a powerful episode of his groundbreaking series *Atlanta*, rapper and actor Donald Glover showed his character receiving counseling and acknowledging his fear of vulnerability.

Yet it's still a widespread belief in the Black community and beyond that Black people, and particularly Black men, don't go to counseling. That they don't need it. That they don't deserve it.

The conventional thinking has been that therapy is for those who are rich, sick, and white. In reality, to seek therapy, you just have to realize you are worthy of health and hope, that you are deserving of a safe place where you can acknowledge, examine, and emerge from your pain.

Black men, taking care of your heart, bettering your life, is part of your divine birthright. Black men, you are indeed worthy.

It's true that Black men don't go to therapy if they fear they will be shamed and blamed, or if they believe they will not be heard. But when they summon the courage to peer inside themselves, or their hurting gets so overwhelming they can no longer ignore it, Black men will not only seek out therapy, but will go and flourish from it.

A therapist might have to cut off her Black male client mid-sentence because he wants to keep talking long after the session is over, like the first time Courtney went to see Dr. K. Her patient may want to move up his appointment because he has so much to wade through and can't wait to share. I know from my own practice that once Black men discover a place where they are welcomed, where they can sit and not be judged, where they can share their ingenuity to survive without having to dam their tears, they will make an appointment, show up for it, and never want to leave.

THE GIFT OF TIME

Therapy can be a vital tool on the road to self-discovery, creating a haven where Black men can bring to the surface conversations that they've been quietly having with themselves their entire lives.

Still, before any of us can figure out how and why we hurt, we must acknowledge our hurt in the first place. If

you worry you are going to be called weak for simply being
human, if you fear you're going to be labeled lame or a
"punk," or you will be dismissed or mocked, you're not going
to admit that you've been injured, let alone seek out someone to help you salve your wounds.

Throughout the history of this nation, Black men have
often been denied the traditional markers of manhood by a
society that accosted their families, and literally hung and
castrated them in a twisted, racist rite meant to terrorize
Black people and uphold the lie and illusion of white supremacy, dominance, and tyranny. To maintain their dignity in
the face of such brutality, many often denied their emotional
or even physical pain. But when Black men are given the
chance to open up, whether in a therapist's office, on a golf
course, or in a barber's chair, thoughts and feelings can flow.

A few years ago, I was invited to facilitate a conference
in Denver, Colorado. It was a gathering of accomplished
Black men who were top executives, seasoned professionals,
and all-around pillars of their communities. I was the only
woman in attendance. Even the servers were male.

The setting was a generic ballroom in a generic hotel,
but the reason for the gathering was wrenching. Yet another
video of a Black man being executed by police was in heavy
rotation, the latest in a nauseating loop of Black death
that seemed to endlessly flood our social media feeds and
screens.

These Black men in their tailored suits, letters of professional and educational distinction trailing their names,
had gathered to deal with another gut punch reminder that
Black life could be snuffed out in a second, and not even
the biggest street protests in American history could stop

it. The police just kept on killing. So they came together in that hotel to discuss Black trauma. They came together to discuss their trauma.

I started out tentatively.

"Hello. I'm Dr. Robin."

My introduction was met with polite applause. I knew I had to explain why I, a woman, was there in this all-male space. I realized I might have to convince more than a few skeptics why a therapist even needed to be present. I acknowledged the elephant in the room.

"I know this is holy ground, and you don't know if I'm safe yet. But I recognize that it is an honor to be here, that I am one woman among all of you. I am not a spy. I am your ally. You can take it to the bank that I won't kiss and tell. If you hear something from this room on the street, you better look around to see who else you told, because rest assured, it wasn't me."

There was soft laughter. Then one by one, men began to rise, peeling back layers as they took the mic.

One told of social anxiety he'd begun to experience, turning interactions in the office into herculean tasks. Another talked about how helpless he felt every time his teenage son left the house, worried that he might have an encounter with a store clerk, security guard, or cop that could end in tragedy.

It went on, a kind of call and response as one man offered a glimpse into his soul followed by his brothers yelling out affirmations or saluting his candor with applause. Occasionally, after a particularly poignant anecdote, a tender space emerged where everyone sat in respectful silence, nodding their heads, saying nothing at all and there were tears. We all wept.

Our forty-five-minute discussion stretched to sixty minutes, then ninety. Finally, after three hours, a hotel employee nervously signaled that we had to wrap it up. Another event was scheduled, and we'd paid to have the room for a much shorter block of time.

The conference had become like one of my therapy sessions where I had a Black male patient who felt he was being heard for the first time. No one wanted to go. And that offers an important lesson. When we who love or counsel Black men give them the chance to talk about their mental and emotional challenges, it is important not to rush them. It is imperative that we just listen and let them know they have time to figure out whether this environment is worthy of their story, and to discern if this space is deserving of their effort.

Offering Black men time is in itself a profound gesture because they are so often dismissed or ignored. It is a deeply meaningful act to give Black men the grace to use their innate wisdom to determine whether or not this space, this book, this initiative is worthy of their leaning in.

That's why my first words at that gathering in Denver acknowledged that I had to show myself worthy of their attention. They understood that I knew something about their duress, that I had a scholarly expertise, but that didn't mean I deserved hours of their day. They had the right to test me.

In that gathering, everyone chose to make room for each man's story to unfold in all its complexity. We ignored our smart phones and the clock on the wall to allow those narratives to take whatever twists and turns that were necessary.

You deserve the time to ask questions and to look for answers. Therapy can grant you the space and privacy you need to shake those loose. But first, you have to trust it.

NOWHERE TO LAY MY BURDEN DOWN

Black people's reluctance to seek out therapy has been fueled in part by a distrust of the health care system. A 2020 survey conducted by the Kaiser Family Foundation and the online platform *The Undefeated* found that almost 6 in 10 Black Americans had little to no confidence that the U.S. health care system would look out for their communities.*

That same wariness kept many Black men and women from receiving the COVID-19 vaccine in the midst of a global health crisis. The reasons for this suspiciousness are understandable.

The year 2022 was the fiftieth anniversary of the news report that exposed the Tuskegee Experiment, one of the most notorious examples of how the medical system debases Black bodies. In that infamous project that began in the early 1930s, hundreds of Black men were used to study the effects of syphilis and denied treatment even after it was discovered that penicillin was an effective remedy.

As powerfully described by Dr. Arline T. Geronimus in her book *Weathering: The Extraordinary Stress of Ordinary Life in an Unjust Society*, "In members of groups that are othered and demeaned, who must struggle for validation or success against strong headwinds, a set of physiological pathways are chronically activated that can lead to cardiovascular

---

* "New Nationwide Poll by the Kaiser Family Foundation and The Undefeated Reveals Distrust of the Health Care System Among Black Americans." Kaiser Family Foundation, Oct. 13, 2020. https://www.kff.org/racial-equity-and-health-policy/press-release/new-nationwide-poll-by-the-kaiser-family-foundation-and-the-undefeated-reveals-distrust-of-the-health-care-system-among-black-americans/.

disease, cancer, accelerated aging, weakened immune systems, and other life-threatening vulnerabilities."

Numerous studies have also found that Black people are perceived to have a higher threshold for pain and not given the same treatment for it as their white peers. A 2016 article in the *Proceedings of the National Academy of Sciences of the United States of America* reported that a significant number of whites, including medical students and residents, thought Blacks and whites were physiologically different, and such bigoted notions led to Black patients not receiving the prescriptions they required, and the overmedicating and prescribing to white people, causing the opioid crisis in white America.

When it comes to mental well-being, Black people are not the only community in the United States whose needs are inadequately addressed. Our society overall does a poor job of addressing psychological and emotional health, failing to recognize that depression, anxiety, and various mental disorders can be as devastating or life threatening as a diagnosis of diabetes or cancer. And Black men's specific neglect by the health care system may not always be intentionally racist or malevolent. Many Black boys and men feel pressured to fit into the straitjacket that is society's definition of masculinity, and so a teacher, a coach, and even some medical professionals might miss the cues to their mental distress.

A depressed man, for instance, might not necessarily curl up catatonic in a corner. Instead, he might work round the clock, to the point when he is too tired to feel. The bus driver you see every morning might outwardly appear friendly and just fine. But he might have to claw through anxiety just to make his way out the front door. And you might only get a hint that the studious middle school student you mentor is struggling emotionally when you notice his sliding grades.

However Black men's pain shows up, and whether it is deliberately ignored or simply misunderstood, it is easy to see why in the face of such callousness and disinterest, Black men have often chosen to simply take all their worries to God or to the lonely abyss of nowhere.

DEMONS AND THE HOLY GHOST

Since Black people were first brought by force to this continent four centuries ago, faith has been our anchor, a beacon and foundation that enabled us to endure the abject terror of living in a world that denied our humanity. We learned to whisper our troubles in prayer, or to shout them out on Sunday, releasing our agony in the name of the Father, the Son, and the Holy Ghost.

We were taught all that was wrong and unjust in the world would be made right and fair in the great by-and-by. And today many Black men and women continue to hold on to that belief, often cloaking their struggles in euphemisms.

"I'm too blessed to be stressed! God's got me and I've got this."

"I'm blessed and highly favored."

There are Black men who brandish affirmations like amulets, warding off despair about their earthly worries. And those mantras, like prayer, certainly do have merit. They can buoy your mood, get you through a hard day, or just help you hang on and inch forward from one moment to the next.

You may also ignore the toll life's challenges take on you mentally because you are simply too tired to take on one more thing. But no one gets through life unscathed, and self-care is a necessity and a requirement. Living in denial of what you are feeling and experiencing actually leads to more stress and erodes the potential to find resources and remedies to transform trauma and adversity into purpose and power. Ignoring our internal reality eventually leaves us weak, fragile, and ill.

We all have a right—given by our creator—to experience our full humanity. That means recognizing that the holes that emerge in our lives when we lose a loved one, suffer a broken heart, or endure a setback contribute to our ultimately becoming a fully developed human being. Every experience and all behavior has meaning and purpose.

I know that relationships, that racism, that life can be exhausting. But when we take the time to acknowledge our emotional pain, we can catch a second wind. We can redirect all the energy it takes to suppress what we feel and ignore where we hurt to create, imagine, and love. That is nothing less than a holy endeavor.

And so, it's time for a different kind of altar call, one that encourages Black men to use every available tool to help care for yourselves, and to purge the pain that blocks your joy. You can be both blessed and stressed. And therapy can help you find your way, breath by breath, and step by step.

PRACTICING WHAT YOU PREACH

I have not only provided therapy. I have received and benefited from it as well.

That surprises some folks. Just as many people don't expect a celebrity like Courtney to struggle, there are those who assume a psychologist, with all my education and training, sails through life calmly, able to easily navigate any rough seas.

But like everyone, I trip and fall. I am willing to acknowledge my emotional battles, because if I'm inviting my Black brothers to be vulnerable and to tell their truths, I must be open and share my own.

I first went to counseling when I was a teenager, struggling to get over a romance that ended unhappily. Later as a psychology student, I was encouraged to seek therapy; it made sense to avail myself of the type of treatment I was going to make a career out of offering to others.

I've always found it profoundly helpful to have someone I could talk to who was impartial in a way friends or family members couldn't always be. But there have been particular moments when having that neutral sounding board was especially meaningful.

About a decade ago, I began to feel separated from myself, caught between how the world saw me and what I knew deep inside to be true. I'd started working with Black inner-city kids who were being detained at a youth center in Philadelphia. And from the very first day, it was clear that I was being labeled. The social workers and security guards saw me walk in, heard me speak, and thought, "You've got to be joking."

"You don't understand these kids," their shade seemed to say. "You all have nothing in common. Go back to wherever you came from and work with people like you."

It was painful to once again feel as falsely labeled and as misunderstood as many of the detained youth. I felt I didn't fit in anywhere though I knew intuitively that, as a loving human being, I belonged everywhere. It was during that time I stumbled upon a poem called "Love After Love" by the great West Indian writer Derek Walcott.

> The time will come
> when, with elation
> you will greet yourself arriving
> at your own door, in your own mirror,
> and...
> You will love again the stranger who was your self.

Those words let me know that, before I sought other people's validation, it was essential that I understood and loved myself.

That poem was medicine. It reassured me that I didn't need to wait for someone else to be glad or excited that I was in the room. I could be elated when I looked in the mirror and greeted myself. There was something radical about that, about understanding that however vulnerable or damaged I might be, I was enough. I felt freedom, and a little bit of peace.

Seeing and embracing myself, even when that confidence was at times fleeting, became the most transformative action I ever took in my life.

That's the self-discovery that can happen through therapy. Yes, Black man, you're upset. Too often when you arrive at the door, people are terrified. They peek from behind it or slam it shut. But you can find solace in your own embrace. No one knows you better. No one loves you more. You can open the door and celebrate that it is you standing there.

That was the message Courtney began to receive when he connected with Dr. K, a therapist with whom he felt safe. Someone who gave him the time and eventually the tools to see his story in full. At first, Courtney didn't know that he needed to talk. Then, for all his eloquence, when he tried to make sense of his father's suicide, he didn't know how to speak. But Courtney didn't need to find his voice. He just needed to sit still long enough that he could finally hear it. Therapy, with the gentle guiding hand of Dr. K, helped him do that.

Therapy enables the building of a relationship that has seldom been available to most Black men. It can create a place where you can say anything and everything, where you can unpack and dismantle, whisper and shout, reflect or rage. It's a space to be dizzy, to be in chaos, to be the creator of a universe in which you can discern what is giving you an advantage, and discard what tears you down.

Our loved ones and peers have their own experiences that they filter life through. That can lead them to have many opinions. But therapy is a space where there is no judgment. When you judge yourself, you must render a verdict. You are good or bad. You have failed or triumphed. With a trusted therapist, you create a partnership where you can explore everything because you judge nothing.

Then you can make choices that are truly yours. You don't have to adhere to low expectations imposed by a system that is hostile to Black men at best, engaged in sabotage at worst. You don't have to embody who your parents say you are or who you'll become. You can choose how you move for yourself, by yourself, making the best decisions for you, all on your own.

Who's that stranger? Who is the person you were before racism happened to you? Before you internalized ideals of masculinity that portray white men as swaggering cowboys and Black men as menacing thugs? Who were you before society and family, poverty or struggle chipped away at your self-esteem?

To reconnect with yourself and to love who you are is not narcissistic. It's wholistic. To embrace yourself, holes and all, is the mission of your soul.

A GOOD WORD

In recent years, therapy has become more accessible and acceptable to Black men, especially as their brothers, from celebrities to CEOs, gang members to labor organizers, speak up about what it means to be a Black man in America and the role counseling can play in coping with challenges. Their truth telling lets others know that their pain has purpose, and that their emotional exploration is vital to a broader conversation about mental health and well-being.

But just as Courtney initially struggled to find the right counselor, many who are interested in therapy do not know how to begin. The first step is to find someone you trust enough to let them know that you hurt, and then to ask them if they know anyone who's helped other hurting people. That's what Courtney did when he let his massage therapist know that he had suffered a loss that was causing him a searing pain.

Word of mouth isn't worth much if it comes from just anyone. You want recommendations from people who you see doing their work. People who you know are honing their own emotional muscles, growing themselves up.

A referral from another Black man isn't essential, but it can be more reassuring as you begin your own mental health journey. When you hear personal testimonials from a peer about how therapy gave them the insights to work out issues in a worthy marriage, the conviction to adopt a child, or the strength to leave a toxic workplace, it can put you more at ease. That is also why it is so important for Black men who have sought counseling to share their experiences, to lift the stigma that lingers and widen the circle of healing.

A primary physician or other trusted medical professional is also a potentially good resource. An internist refers patients for all kinds of care, from dermatology to podiatry, so if your ailment is emotional, your physician should be able to help you find a psychiatrist or psychologist to consult with.

Of course, you then have to figure out how to pay for it. Medical care in the United States can be prohibitively expensive, and many Americans do not have insurance; this includes roughly 11% of Black Americans, according to a 2017 factsheet from the American Psychiatric Association. Then, even if you do have coverage for health care, you may not have the spare cash to cover a stream of co-payments. And many mental health professionals do not accept insurance at all. But fortunately, many cities have community resources to help fill the void.

In October 2022, President Joe Biden announced that his administration would give funds to increase the number of Certified Community Behavioral Health Clinics, which offer around-the-clock mental health support, regardless of ability to pay. He has also said that there is federal funding available to raise the number of mental health counselors at the nation's schools, and to help young people get emotional support through telehealth services.

College counseling centers often have clinicians who are accumulating the hours necessary for their training—don't sell them short because they are still working toward their certifications. It means the fee may be on a sliding scale or treatment may be free. Community mental health centers are also an option, often offering free or very-low-cost care.

There are also online resources that can help you find a professional who specializes in treating people in Black communities, which leads to another frequently asked question.

DOES YOUR THERAPIST NEED TO BE BLACK?

Many people assume your mental health professional should be of the same ethnic background or gender as you. In my opinion, it's not wholly necessary. People have said to me, "Dr. Robin, I'm an ordained minister. So it's important that my therapist is a Christian."

I greet those questions and statements with the same response.

"If you needed heart surgery," I ask, "would you be seeking a Black, Christian cardiothoracic surgeon? Or would you just want a doctor who could get you off the table alive?"

Let me be clear: I don't mean to undermine the need to engage with educators, employers, and health professionals who are culturally competent—or to use a term coined by my colleague and friend Dr. Howard Stevenson, racially literate. Cultural fluency helps cut down the time you have to spend translating particular experiences. You don't want the microaggressions you experience because of your skin color to be downplayed. If you're religious, you might be concerned that someone of a different faith, or who has no faith at all, won't understand you. You don't want to be encouraged to consider divorce, for instance, when your religion maintains divorce is wrong.

Still, if you focus on appearances and categories, you may miss out on the person who's best equipped to help you do the work you need to do. Courtney, a Black man who is Christian, found his synergy with Dr. K, a white, Jewish woman. It's the guidance and safety that matters, not the package that it comes in. What we really want in treatment, and what Black men deserve, is someone who sees you and wants to accompany you on your wellness journey.

Can you help me? Do you get me? Where can I find healing? Those are the questions you need to ask, whether you are entrusting your money, your physical health, or your mind to someone else. You don't necessarily need a therapist whose experiences most mirror your own, or who wants to issue edicts about how you should live your life. Rather, you want to find that someone who is worthy of, and willing to make room for, your narrative. You want to find that person who understands their job is to help you get the mud in your mind to settle, so the water can run clear.

"Is there anything I should know?"

"Where does it hurt?"

Those are the questions that Black men are entitled to ask themselves and each other. Those are the questions all those who love and care about Black men should ask them as well.

QUICK TIPS FOR WORKING WITH MENTAL HEALTH PROFESSIONALS

✳ **Get a referral.** Your primary physician can help connect you to a professional counselor.

✳ **Tell a friend.** Ask a peer if they have a recommendation, particularly if they have sought counseling for themselves.

✳ **Seek out free services.** If you are worried about cost, look for a counseling center at the nearest university, or seek out a community health program where fees for services may be on a sliding scale, or free.

✳ **Look online.** Some good resources include the Boris Lawrence Henson Foundation, founded by actress Taraji P. Henson: https://resourceguide.borislhensonfoundation.org/.

✳ **Be open.** The best therapist for you may not be the same race, religion, or gender. They don't need to be. You just need to be comfortable and believe that they will provide a safe haven where you can share your story and fully explore your feelings.

✳ **Where does it hurt?** Those who love, or counsel, you should grant you the time to sort out whether you are ready to give voice to your experiences, and if they are the right one for you to tell. If they are—and you are—let them ask you about your hurt, and you can ask them for their willingness to listen patiently.

CHAPTER 3

(Black) Men Don't Cry

"The lion's story will never be known as long as the hunter is the one to tell it."

—AFRICAN PROVERB

If I didn't know how to find a therapist, or "do" therapy, I definitely didn't know how to catch a dream. Who knew that was even a thing? Dr. K had just given me the assignment without any direction. I had to figure out how to capture my dreams on my own.

The New School is a research college in New York City known for its progressive teachings about everything from social sciences to design, so if there was any place that had a course on something as unconventional as capturing your dreams, I knew that was it. There wasn't any Google then. I picked up a school catalog, and sure enough, Dr. Gayle Delaney was teaching a workshop based on her book *Breakthrough Dreaming*.

I was onstage nearly every night for seven years, but to take the class and really absorb what I was learning, I decided for the first time to take a break. It wasn't some big departure announced in the Arts Section of the *New York Times*. I just told my stage manager that I was going to be coming down with "something" and would be out for a long weekend.

"I think I'm going to have a cold"—*cough*—"in about a month." *Cough, cough.*

"Okay, Court," he said. "I've got you." *Wink, wink.*

My understudy filled in wonderfully while I made my way down to Greenwich Village that weekend to take the course. Our class was a hodgepodge of psychology majors, new age enthusiasts, and folks like me who were just searching.

Many psychologists and cultures have detailed the significance of dreams. Some believe they are our way of tapping into our subconscious longings while others think they are a portal that allows us to transcend the boundary between the earthly world and the afterlife.

Dr. Delaney talked about how the symbols, experiences, and places that come to us as we sleep can give us a road map to dealing with challenges we encounter when we're awake. But when she asked how many of us remembered our dreams, hardly any hands went up. She had to teach us how to do it.

"I want you to put a pencil, note pad, and flashlight by your bed," Dr. Delaney said. "Then, write the first thing you can recall when you wake up, whether it's a couple hours into your sleep or after a full night's rest. At first it may be hard because many of us put no stock in dreams, so there's no reason to hold on to them. But once you make the effort, it will become easier. You're training your mind. Challenge yourself."

I picked up a couple eight-by-ten-inch sketch books from an art store near my apartment, scrounged around my kitchen for a flashlight and the nub of a Number 2 pencil, and got to work.

Dr. Delaney said, ideally, we should be in bed by 9:00 or 9:30. Typically you'd sleep solidly until 2:00 in the morning, and then from 2:00 to, say, 6:00 a.m., you move deep into your REM cycle. That's when your most vivid dreams begin.

At first, because I was so used to waking up and immediately starting the day, the memories of my dreams wafted away like smoke. But I began to ask myself, "Where was I?" as soon as I opened my eyes in the morning, forcing myself to lie still as the sun seeped through the blinds.

With Dr. Delaney's direction and a new routine, my dreams began to flicker before me like an Instagram reel. I jotted down all that I could remember. And by the time I saw Dr. K again, I had thirty-five dreams to discuss, complete with titles!

"You told me to go get my dreams, Dr. K, and I've got thirty-five!" I said triumphantly.

Just like the first time we met, when I tripped all over myself spilling my thoughts and feelings, Dr. K had to slow me down.

"Bring me your most powerful dream, Courtney, not all of them," she said. "We'll go from there."

That following Tuesday, I returned to the show, but I remained diligent. *Six Degrees* was only ninety minutes long, so we'd be done by 9:30 and the cast would sometimes get a bite to eat. But not me. I'd grab a snack, run home, walk my dog, Bottom, then hop into bed, knowing I was already slightly behind Dr. Delaney's sleep schedule. Before long, I had enough dream-filled notebooks to fill an entire shelf.

————

Looking back, I guess I was always my mama's boy.

Like most families where siblings gravitate more toward one parent than the other, my sister and I paired off. Cecilie was like my dad, with the same inquisitiveness and desire to debate. Meanwhile, I was closer to our mother, pensive, quiet, and enjoying nothing more than curling up with a good book to read.

Now trust me, nobody loved my dad more than me. I followed him everywhere. When he worked on that van of his, painted the color of sunshine, I'd be right beside him, handing him the tools. When he picked up fertilizer from the hardware store or visited one of his friends, I was always game to tag along. And in many ways, I was the stereotypical "boy's boy," excelling in Pee Wee and Little League sports before becoming the anchor of my high school's varsity teams. I would have added lacrosse or soccer to my regimen but there simply weren't enough hours in the day.

Still, it was my mother who really got me. She knew I was a sensitive child at a time when sensitive wasn't the thing to be, not for a Black boy who excelled in sports, not for any boy really. She gave me the space to be who I was. That understanding and emotional connection drew us together.

I cried easily. I boo-hooed when Marie Hollis told me she didn't want to be my Valentine in the seventh grade, and I poured out a whole bucket of tears when the Detroit Lions lost the playoffs just a couple games shy of making it to the Super Bowl. And don't let me hear the speech Glynn Turman gave in tribute to his fallen friend "Cochise," played by Lawrence Hilton Jacobs in the film classic *Cooley High*. Every time I watched it on television after school, I'd go outside, sit on the grass, and sob like a baby.

It was a day like that, when I was deep in my feelings, that I did something I'd never done before and would never do again and that was to curse at my father. It was because he made a joke about Rana.

Rana was one of our two dogs. In contrast to Pepper, our tiny terrier, Rana was a majestic reddish-brown shepherd. By the time

I was a teenager, Rana was slowing down, refusing to chase the ball when I threw it, sleeping a lot more, and slightly dragging her left leg. I saw what was happening, but it was unthinkable to imagine a time when Rana wouldn't be with us.

That's why when Dad started cracking jokes one afternoon about putting Rana to sleep, I temporarily lost my mind.

"How can you make a joke like that?" I screamed. "That's not f—funny!"

I ran up the stairs in tears. I heard my mother's voice. She was trying to calm my father down.

"Leslie," Dad said quietly, "he can't talk to me like that!"

A couple minutes later, I heard my mother walking up the stairs. She opened my bedroom door. At first, she was quiet.

"Oh, man," I thought, still angry at my dad but now also realizing the stupidity of what I'd done. When my mother just stood there looking at you without talking, you knew you were in trouble.

"Son," she said finally. "You will go downstairs and apologize to your father."

"I'm. Sorry," I stammered between sobs. "But. Daddy. Was joking. About putting Rana to sleep."

"I know," she said. "But you know you can't talk to your father like that."

I was sixteen years old, but when I went back downstairs, I leaped into my father's arms like I was a toddler, still crying, but now so sorry.

I just hugged my dad, repeating over and over, I'm so sorry, Daddy, I'm so sorry! All that was left to say was the simple, painful truth. "It's okay," he said. "I know it hurts, but Rana is sick. We're going to have to put her to sleep."

I realize now that having to contemplate Rana's twilight

probably crushed Dad even more than me. I'd played with her every day, but it was Dad who'd trained her and taken her to get her shots. She was much more his dog than mine. Now he had to make the unimaginable decision to put her down to end her suffering.

I didn't get then how the man who was everything to me could joke about something so awful, but now I understand. He couldn't allow himself to sink into his pain. He couldn't allow himself to be vulnerable. So he made a joke instead. That was his way of enduring an unbearable situation.

When you grow up in a household, you know where you can go and where you can't, what rooms you can enter and what rooms to stay out of. My father never told me not to cry, but I knew instinctively that was not his way. He didn't even break down when he took Rana to the vet for the last time, or when we buried her. I looked up to my father, but my mother was my mirror, where I could see myself because I knew that she saw me.

There was only so far Dad could go with me emotionally because to go deeper would mean possibly facing questions that he wasn't ready to answer. Like how bad did it hurt to have never known his mother? How lonely did he feel growing up with a foster father he couldn't always rely on? Dad couldn't give me that space because he was locked in his own battle.

And as emotional as I was as a kid, as much as I was my mother's son, I also understood there was a time to be disciplined and in control. We lived in a world where, as Black people, if we tangled with the police or just a random white stranger, we might be hurt, or even killed. Like most Black parents, ours made sure we realized there were rules to follow and lines you didn't cross. That training started at home so we could shift into autopilot when we were out and about in the world.

"Court, your dad is on the porch calling for you," my friends would say if I'd stayed outside when the streetlights came on. "Is there anything we can do?"

They were just glad it was my dad standing on that porch and not theirs.

"No," I'd say, bracing for that belt I was about to feel on my behind for being out past curfew. "Leave me alone. I'm in trouble."

That didn't happen too often. I knew when to play and when to work hard. I knew how to walk a straight line, and how to make my family proud.

My tearful downpours were the rare times when I let my guard down. And the older I got, the less I cried. I had business to handle. I had things to do. I couldn't afford to be vulnerable.

And then I learned how to do Shakespeare.

———

During my junior year at Harvard, I was part of a show called *Lulu* at the American Repertory Theater. I was more behind the scenes, manipulating the boom mike in the play, which simulated a film noir, and speaking just a few lines. But I got to work with the great actress Cathy Slade, and at the end of the show's run, as related previously, she suggested I try out for Shakespeare & Company, a theater troupe with apprenticeship grants that would allow some who were selected to attend for free.

I expected to audition in a hall or theater. Instead, I found myself doing a monologue in the kitchen of a century-old house on Edith Wharton's estate while some of the instructors chopped carrots and prepared dinner. It was odd to say the least, but I made the cut. I told my girlfriend about the experience when I got back home, and she decided to audition as well. A few days later we were both in, and that summer we boarded a bus and headed for the woods.

On one of our first nights, we were told we were going to do a week-long clown workshop with Clownmaster Merry Conway. She immediately threw us into "the deep end" with an exercise called, "Circle of Fire."

"Is that some campfire thing where we all light matches and sing in the moonlight?" I thought. We were in the woods after all.

It wasn't that.

Our group was going to form a circle in the dance studio where we did our voice classes, leaving just enough space for someone to walk in or out. Then each of the apprentices would take turns standing in the center of the ring. In the span of a few minutes, we had to make the group laugh and cry. Then we'd exit, and the next person would step up.

The only ground rules were no vulgarity or cursing. So we spent an hour getting ready, pulling prosthetic noses out of prop boxes and trying on toupees. "This is gonna be fun," I said to myself.

Man, I'd never been more wrong. Can I tell you that when you stand in front of a group not knowing what you're doing, not only is it not fun, but five minutes is endless?

Someone would toss out a corny joke that landed like a pile of concrete. Someone else did an emotional scene that came across overly sentimental. Nobody was laughing, and there wasn't a tear in sight.

Finally, the last person walked out of the circle with her head hanging down and our instructor told us what we already knew. Yes, she said, we were all terrible. And that's what we had to face. That's what we had to claim.

That, she explained, was the secret to moving an audience. There was no shame in failure. You just had to acknowledge it. Merry called it, "Taking the Bead." When you did, that's the moment you broke open. You and that woman in the first row could burst out laughing together because you both knew you'd bombed in the scene before. Or maybe she'd feel so sorry for you, she'd teeter on the brink of tears and let them loose after your next monologue.

Most of us feel embarrassed when we fail. But when we miss the mark in public, that's when we're most raw and human. That's an emotion everyone can relate to. And when you mess up and own it instead of trying to run and hide, nobody can bring you down. Then, you're free.

That lesson has stuck with me for forty years. But in those early weeks of summer, I didn't get it, and I just wanted to go home.

I tried to latch on to my girlfriend.

"Would you stop it?" she said to me one afternoon, exasperated. "I've got my own problems, and we are here with fourteen other people! We have to all support each other!"

Everyone—the teachers, the other apprentices—knew I was struggling. Each day was more wrenching than the one before.

One of our next tasks involved a classic Shakespeare & Company exercise—"Dropping In" a scene (or an entire play). Two actors would sit directly across from each other, interlocking knees, and a third and/or a fourth person would "drop in" the line, whispering them in their ears with repetitions, suggestions, and subtle subliminal meanings. It was an exhausting, exhilarating experience that would often leave the actors breathless, giggling, and/or crying uncontrollably. For example, if we were dropping in a scene from *Hamlet*, reciting one of the most famous pairing of words in the English language, it would go something like this: "To be," your facilitator would say. "What does that mean, to be? What does it mean to you, Courtney? Have you ever thought about not being?"

I wanted to be back home in Cambridge, far away from here.

Just as upsetting was the fact that I was having a hard time with the dialogue in *Romeo and Juliet,* the scene my scene-partner and I prepared all summer to perform.

There's something that many people may not realize about Shakespeare. His words flow like a heartbeat, ten beats to a line. Every punctuation mark means something, from the semicolon to the comma. When there is a beat less or a beat more, it means there's a particular emotional punch embedded in the words. And for whatever reason, I just couldn't get the rhythm.

Then one day, near the end of the program, I was rehearsing the balcony scene.

" 'O blessed, blessed night. I am afeard, / Being in night, all this is but a dream, / Too flattering-sweet to be substantial.' "

And it happened.

The dam burst. All the emotion packed in that line, in that scene, surged through me like an electric current.

I have no idea what the key was, but I no longer resisted being vulnerable. Instead of worrying about messing up, or being embarrassed, I allowed myself to really feel the emotional depth of the words I was saying. From that day on, I could move an audience to tears by reading from the phone book if I wanted to. Whatever the moment called for, I would feel it in my marrow. And it wasn't rehearsed. It wasn't mimicry. It was real.

When I returned to Harvard, I marinated in what I'd learned. And by the time I returned to the Shakespeare theater program the following summer, my instincts were as sharp as a knife.

This time, we were to perform Shakespeare's *Comedy of*

Errors. I wanted to be one of the two sets of twins, whose travails and near misses form the comedic arc, but our director wanted me to be the sad old man, Egeon, who introduces the play's backstory.

I didn't like that. I wanted to make folks laugh and have fun. I sulked about what I thought was my miscasting after every rehearsal.

When it was finally showtime, we held our first performance outdoors for the local community on a warm but overcast day.

I hobbled out to the stage.

" 'Here's the story,' " I began, my back bent, my voice deep. " 'Two twins get lost and shipwrecked.... And I just want to find my family.' " I punctuated that last word, "family," with a heartrending wail.

There is a time, in a play or on a sound stage, when you, the cast, and everyone who's watching move as one. It's as if all of you together tap into the same invisible frequency. It's what I finally felt in *Six Degrees* after the first few frustrating months. It's what I experienced with Mary Alice, James Earl Jones, and Frankie Faison when we costarred in *Fences.*

And that's what happened that day in Massachusetts. My opening monologue became a mournful song, and when I recited those words, the whole mood in that clearing changed.

At the end of my scene, I put my hands up in the air, and the sun broke through and shone down on all of us. The audience and my castmates literally gasped.

Growing up, as a top student, I was taught to be cerebral, to figure everything out in my head. As I got older, I became more my father's son, stoic and in control. But performing Shakespeare forced me to make a shift. I had to give in to the truth that there are some things you can't figure out. Sometimes all you can do is be still and just let the feelings come, not when you want them to, not if you want them to, but whenever they're ready.

That was the kind of acceptance and patience Dr. K hoped I could find in my day-to-day life. Therapy was helping me get back to the little boy who wasn't afraid to cry, to connect emotionally offstage the way I did when I was on. She wanted me to live like the actor who felt so deeply during a scene, it seemed he had the power to part clouds and summon the sun.

Slowly, I was leaving behind the Courtney who wanted to run away after his father's suicide, who mentally flipped a coin to decide whether to take a particular apartment, try out for a role, or end a relationship. Instead of worrying about being exposed as less than perfect, I was beginning to recognize that my failings were helping me to grow up. And even if I didn't immediately understand the lesson, the answers would eventually come. I just had to let the mud settle in the water, and the water become clear.

As I burrowed deeper and deeper into my dreams, Dr. K said we should increase our schedule and see each other two or three times a week. I would have gone to see her every single day if I'd been able to, and unlike many of my Black brothers, also hurting, also searching, I had the income and the insurance that enabled me to see her as often as I needed. It was a blessing.

To be or not to be vulnerable. That was the question.

I was choosing "to be."

Where Do You Hurt?

When was the last time you saw yourself? Have you ever? Who were you before the first person told you to "man up" or "boys don't cry," before you took that to heart, held your breath, and decided that you would never cry again?

Tending to your emotional health means acknowledging that you've had experiences and encounters that caused you pain. Then, the next essential question is, Where does it hurt? Does your fragile heart make it harder to commit to a romantic partner? Does your broken confidence make you quick tempered, or prevent you from pursuing a goal or job or credential you'd like to attain?

You are beginning to peel back the layers of yourself. One question leads to another. And the next query that should be high on the list for every Black man is, Who am I?

To find the answer, you will first have to look in the mirror.

I'm not talking about the piece of glass hanging above the bathroom sink, but the reflection in your mind's eye. For too many Black boys and men, your mirror is distorted, reflecting a toxic, angry caricature, or a person unworthy of love, neither of which is who you are.

But that mirror has been warped and shaped by a society that doesn't know anything about you or has its own motives for making sure you do not see or appreciate your essence. Once that cracked glass is repaired, once that mirror is scrubbed and polished, you can gaze upon yourself in all your glory. When the mirror reflects who you really are, and not someone else's twisted misrepresentation, your whole, complicated, yet worthy self will be revealed to you, perhaps for the first time.

Our elders have passed down their wisdom through the ages, encapsulated in stories, in songs, and in sayings that distill profound truths into a few sharp words.

"God don't like ugly."

"Every shut eye ain't sleep."

Then there are the African proverbs. One that I especially love warns that the lion's story will never be known as long as the hunter is the one doing the telling.

It's similar to another old saying about how history is written by the winners. But I find the African passage more resonant, not just because it descends from our ancestors but because when it comes to Black men, the architects of a system that has abused them for centuries—the literal hunters—have been in charge of their narrative for far too long.

When I worked at the Youth Study Center in Philadelphia, I watched the young, mostly Black, youth go in front of judges with their slouching pants and their hair uncombed. I knew from my own experience how easy it was for people to stamp a label on you based on factors as superficial as your appearance. I knew that some of the employees in that very center made up stories about me based on how I looked and spoke, assuming I was just a bourgie do-gooder trying to make myself feel charitable. They grabbed bits and pieces of me, indeed those that were the least meaningful, to form a whole misguided impression.

But their opinions wouldn't impact my life. Unlike a juvenile court judge, they didn't have the power to decide whether I would be locked up for the next five or ten or twenty years. So, when I sat down with these children whose lives were in danger of ending before they truly began, I asked them what they were thinking going into a courtroom with the tops of their underwear poking out.

"I'm doing me, Dr. Robin!" they'd say defiantly. "I'm not changing myself for nobody!"

I realized I had to school them about the hunter.

"Do you know what Wall Street is?" I asked.

Yeah, several responded. It was a place where people sold stocks.

"Well," I continued, "do you know they're getting people to invest in really fancy prisons? And do you know who they're building those prisons for? They're building them for you. They're counting on young men like you filling them up. They have a pipeline that goes from this center right to the Big House, and they're planning for all of you to subsidize their lives, for you to pay for their children's college educations, while you're sitting behind bars rotting."

"So, when you go in front of the judge with your pants sagging down, it's the system that's actually doing you. You're living out a story they wrote to keep you down and to make them rich. But you can make different choices. You have the power to decide whether or not somebody makes millions off your misery."

Every time I framed the situation that way, the swagger would seep out of the room like air in a deflated balloon. Finally, someone would speak.

Were they really building new, fancy prisons? Did they really have a plan?

Yes, I told them. They were literally banking on them not getting out of this system, counting on them not being able to figure out how to become who they were born to be. They were betting that these lion cubs would internalize the fiction written by those who were hunting them and that they would start to believe that sordid story was really their truth.

Society often reduces Black manhood to a handful of stereotypes. There is, of course, the thug, the criminal mold that so many of the young men in that Philadelphia center were contorting themselves to fill. It's the dominant depiction in our popular culture, on the local news, and it's unfortunately embedded in our national psyche.

And then when you move from the gory to the glory, it is the rapper or athlete who is held up as a shimmering example of Black masculinity. Of course, white athletes and music stars also get more attention than they necessarily deserve. Our culture loves celebrities. But white men see themselves reflected in so many places, in so many ways, it's far easier for them to imagine all that they can do and be.

That's not the case for Black men. While society focuses on Jay-Z's billions, Drake's latest hit, or Patrick Mahomes's Super Bowl ring, whose stories aren't being told? Who speaks about all those unsung Black men who are holding it down as fathers and husbands, coaching soccer, looking after their aging parents, or rushing from work to get to their child's dance recital?

Society's mirror doesn't reflect how varied Black men really are, how much you have to share, or how protective and committed you are to your families and communities. That leaves an ugly void that allows lies to obscure your truth. And those stereotypical images can become another prison, determining not only how others see Black boys and men, but too often how you see yourselves. Many of you are locked in and trapped by the confines of hypermasculinity.

THREE FIFTHS OF A MAN?

When we look at the personas of hip hop stars, pop culture gurus, and gridiron heroes, there is a trait that most share. They're not soft. You never see them cry. They stalk the stage, the street corner, or the football field with a defiant strut.

The sexist belief that men are supposed to be hard and infallible is toxic whatever a man's ethnic or racial background because it can keep him from becoming his more evolved self. But like so many double standards in American life, hypermasculinity for Black boys and men is a particularly dangerous double-edged sword.

For a white man, brazenness and bravado make him a beacon of safety. But paint that archetype Black or brown, and he is a threat, the thug who you need to watch out for and the criminal you are justified to attack, lock up, or even kill. The overlay of race makes the white man the one you want in your corner, while Black men are the predators you want to run away from.

Even worse, such a pervasive caricature often makes Black boys and men want to run away from themselves. In a perverse paradox, the same posture and swagger that leads society to target them also draws them adoration, and in that they find a sort of protection. So, many emulate that macho ideal, refusing to be vulnerable, ignoring their more delicate inner selves.

In the eighteenth century, Black people were declared three fifths of a human being to appease racist slave owners, who didn't want their political power diminished because their states were largely populated by people who were owned and treated like chattel. That legal notion was swept away by the Fourteenth Amendment, which made Black people citizens, at least on paper. But Black men and women have been trying to live down the lie that they are less than fully human ever since.

Pushing through and not looking within allows Black men to ignore their untreated trauma, to avoid what they may be afraid to see. Masking fear and fragility has sometimes been and is often key to psychological survival. And certainly, to be vulnerable is to feel exposed. But not allowing yourself to acknowledge and express your hurt can ultimately crush your soul.

It may be up to those who care about Black boys and men to pose the questions that many may be initially reluctant to ask themselves. We live in a world where even Black men who fit society's ideal of success are dodging, ignoring, or bracing for attack. So we can gently cut to the quick. I know that you hurt. Can you tell me how, and where?

You may have to wait for a response. So many Black men don't have the language to capture what it means in the words of the great scholar and historian W. E. B. Du Bois "to be a problem." It may take a while for him to be able to articulate his lived experience, and the fears, worries, and stresses that it provokes. He may struggle to say out loud

what it means to be a little Black boy who is labeled dangerous when he's no more rambunctious than his white playmate, or to be harassed and hunted online and in the street.

Many Black men are struck mute because they find it so
humiliating to be hated by strangers simply because of who
they are. It's like a domestic violence victim who is ashamed
of being abused. They shouldn't feel they have to hide the
truth that their partner is beating them, but their abuser,
and often the broader society, is adept at making them feel
that, somehow, they deserved what they got. They convince
them that the abuse wouldn't happen if they behaved differently or were simply better people.

So, as a result, you might unleash some of your hurt by
yelling and cursing, and that can be a temporary needed
release. But those intermittent, explosive outbursts don't get at
the silent suffering, the scorching pain that comes from walking through the world as a target. Yelling and cursing don't
purge the rage that flows from realizing that, no matter how
much you achieve, how dignified you are, how much respect
you give, there are people who will never see you as equal.

At other times, when Black men do speak out, naysayers
flock to silence them. There is an especially vicious backlash that greets Black men who own how broken or dis-
tressed they are, in large part because when they speak the
truth, they expose the cruel actions of a society that wants to
leave them on the margins, silenced and invisible.

We even saw that happen to President Barack Obama.

Obama dared to make a comment about the senseless
murder of Trayvon Martin, a seventeen-year-old shot to
death on February 26, 2012, by an unrepentant killer who,
to add insult to grievous injury, was also acquitted. Obama

addressed the killing when it happened, and again, in July of the following year, after that shameful verdict was announced.

"You know," he said, according to a transcript of the president's remarks issued by the White House on July 19, 2013, "when Trayvon Martin was first shot, I said that this could have been my son. Another way of saying that is Trayvon Martin could have been me 35 years ago. And when you think about why, in the African American community at least, there's a lot of pain around what happened here, I think it's important to recognize that the African American community is looking at this issue through a set of experiences and a history that doesn't go away."*

It was a very Obama-esque statement, offering context, acknowledging varying perspectives, proposing potential solutions ranging from people examining their own biases to more support being offered to young Black men. He even said the criminal justice system needs to be respected though it hasn't always been fair, and that demonstrations and protests should remain peaceful.

Still, when Obama first declared that Trayvon could have been his child, his opposition went wild. "How dare he?" was the message. His follow-up remarks more than a year later likely sparked a similar reaction. Obama had found the language to say how painful Trayvon's murder had been. They wanted him to eat those words. Part of what Black men grapple with, as they confront a litany of injustices, is an internalized rage that they don't know what to do with. They are ashamed that they have to deal with such

* Barack Obama. "Remarks by the President on Trayvon Martin." Office of the Press Secretary, White House, July 19, 2013. https://obamawhitehouse.archives.gov/the-press-office/2013/07/19/remarks-president-trayvon-martin.

indignities in the first place, and fearful of the ridicule or dismissal they will face if they unveil their anguish.

But to Wake Up!, Show Up!, Grow Up!, Rise Up!™, Black men must first speak up. It is critical that you give a voice to your experiences. A first step is to compassionately listen for your own true voice, and find someone safe to begin sharing your story, and listening to theirs. Not everyone is worthy, deserving or capable of witnessing your sacred journey.

WHAT DO I TELL ME ABOUT ME?

Get quiet. Sit down and ask, "Where do I hurt?"

And then, ponder the internal soundtrack that's stuck on repeat inside your head.

What do I tell me about me? Do I affirm how gifted I am? Do I blame myself for things that were done to me, or put myself down?

After you put a lens on that internal dialogue, ask yourself, Who planted that message? Is that your voice on the tape, or someone else's?

Often, we live out a script without examining its truth or its source. "I just did it because I felt like it," is what we may say about our actions. But there is a reason you are a womanizer, or you break covenants with your children. There is a reason you prioritize your friends over your family or spend money that you don't have.

If you struggle to talk about how you feel, is it because you grew up in a family in which nobody opened up? Or did the folks in your family rage and rail so much, you just shut down?

There are other questions to think about as you begin to excavate your inner world. Ask yourself, What needs did I have? Were they met, and if so, who were the people who met them? While those are questions that can apply to work and grown-up friendships, it's most important to think about those moments from the vantage point of childhood, because that period of your life forms the foundation of all your other relationships.

If you're trying to make do emotionally with very little self-care or support, it's likely that you began, metaphorically, to call crumbs a full meal during childhood. You were likely a little boy when you began to rationalize that while you wished your parents or grandmother would have hugged you more, or asked about your fears without judgment, they did the best they could. But it's critical that you begin to understand that two things can be true at once. Yes, they may have meant well, and yes, they may have given all that they were capable of, and that doesn't mean it was enough. You needed—and deserved—more. It's both-and, not either-or.

Speak about what you begin to discover out loud, to yourself. Get a journal, where you can jot your thoughts down, or even keep notes in your phone. If you like to draw, pull out some paper and sketch a scene; use the appropriate colors to match your feelings. In those private moments, no one else needs to see it. No one else needs to hear it. The goal is to begin to understand how you became you, and how those formative experiences are continuing to shape how you move through your life now.

DON'T ECHO THE HUNTER

Women can play a key role in cracking hypermasculinity's shell and encouraging the men in their lives to voice what's happening in their inner worlds. It's not just fathers, coaches, and home boys who sometimes tell Black men and boys to "man up." Their mothers, sisters, wives, and girlfriends may also say the same. Too often, women desire someone who is strong and unflappable, the rock they can lean on in times of trouble, yet they'll criticize that same man for not being more tender and in tune to their emotional needs.

What invites people to express their feelings, particularly men, is having a partner or a friend who can accept their vulnerability, who lets him know that it's perfectly fine that he doesn't have it all under control. That there is no shame in shedding tears, and that he can't always have all the answers.

It's important for the women in Black men's lives to be a supportive force, and not one that echoes the hunter, putting a million little cracks in the mirror the men they care for hold up to themselves.

I once counseled a couple who, over the years of their marriage, had lashed out at each other in very painful ways, but the husband really wanted to move forward while his wife remained intent on settling scores and having me join in telling her husband what a terrible partner he'd been.

She had suffered severe neglect as a little girl, and now that she was grown and married, she wanted her husband to make it all better. Her anguish originated in her childhood, something her husband had also endured as a child, and as a grown man, he was essentially living on fumes. The more his wife lashed out, the more he shut down, feeling that he was a failure for not being the partner that she wanted him to be.

Through counseling, she came to understand that her husband was not her enemy. She was being haunted and hunted by her history. She needed to look at her own narrative to understand what she was bringing to the table that made her husband's emotional absence so intolerable. It was a liberating moment for both of them when she realized that only she could rescue herself. Each of them had to do their own healing. Then, their mended selves could work together to create a more fulfilling marriage.

Black women, who are also unfairly tasked with society's lie that they are unwaveringly strong, should not expect their sons, brothers, husbands, and fathers to be any more superhuman than they are. I want to encourage women to stand with injured Black men differently. This doesn't mean they should endure mistreatment. It means to be open and awake to the struggles their brothers bring to the table, no matter how uncomfortable it might make them feel as they listen.

When Black women invite Black men to take the floor, when they encourage the boys and men in their lives to expose their whole selves, holes and all, they let them know that they are loved no matter what and enable them to embrace and fully love themselves.

BEAUTY IN THE BROKEN PLACES

There is a cultural assumption that men and women behave fundamentally different when they are on a road trip and they lose their way. The woman, the story goes, usually wants to stop and ask someone for help, while the man refuses to admit defeat, determined to figure it all out on his own.

While that adage has some sexist assumptions, it is a useful metaphor for how men who struggle to acknowledge their emotional wounds can begin to open up. Vulnerability means not being ashamed to ask for directions, whether you get lost driving through an unknown city or feel adrift emotionally. If you don't know the local roads, it makes sense to stop and ask the gas station attendant for guidance. If there's a childhood trauma that haunts you, or an addiction or malaise that is holding you back, it makes sense to seek out a professional counselor, a teammate, or a family elder who will sit, listen, and help you work through it.

Clearly you can't trust any and everybody. Black boys and men often carry an innate suspicion that is not without merit. Sharing your insecurities with the wrong person at work could jeopardize that job you need to pay your bills. If you're a young man in the juvenile detention center and there are supervisors just waiting for the chance to write you up, that person is obviously not someone to confide in.

But you don't need everybody. You don't need ten people. You need just one person who sees you, one person who can be a mirror that reflects back how deserving you are of support, and how even in your brokenness you are beautiful and cherished. You just need one person to whom you can unload that burden that is too heavy to carry by yourself.

That person can be a therapist, like Courtney's Dr. K. But also look at your social circle. Who among your friends is interested and caring enough to hold whatever you share in confidence and to share with you in return?

Reciprocity is important. If you are the only one talking, that doesn't really feel safe. If you run into someone who is dismissive of what you say, who mumbles it will be all right and then ghosts you for the next month, keep moving. Your college roommate may be great to reminisce with about that homecoming party back in the day, but he may not be the best one to tell about the panic attack you had last week when you were waiting at the subway stop trying to get home, or the flashbacks and nightmares that you fend off daily of being sexually abused as a young boy.

It doesn't mean he is a bad person. Maybe he's preoccupied with his own challenges. Maybe your fraternity brother who rushed you off the phone had a deadline to meet, or he just isn't equipped to be the lifesaver you need as you attempt an emotional deep dive. Whatever the backstory, you don't have time to figure out their intentions. Just know this is not your person, at least not in this moment.

Sometimes when we unveil our pain to someone who recoils from it, we give up and resign ourselves to keeping our stories and feelings buried inside. But everyone needs a safe harbor, someone whom he or she can share with. The desire for connection is embedded in our DNA. When you seek out those who will listen to you, those who care, you claim your birthright to community and nurture that kernel of humanity that says you are not meant to be isolated and alone.

So, just like Courtney, it's important to move on from the wrong person, whether it's a therapist who isn't the right fit, or an uninterested friend, but to not give up on the process of finding help. When you find someone willing to take a risk with you, to bare their feelings about what it means to be human, what it means to be Black, what it means specifically to be a Black man, and to listen to your thoughts as well, the search will have been well worth it.

You might find that safe sounding board in a men's group at the local mosque, church, or synagogue. Maybe it's that man or woman you met on a blind date who isn't your romantic soul mate but is a great friend you can talk to. You might gain support from your aunt or great-uncle who you learn has been waiting patiently for the day that you decided on your own to seek their counsel. Or your confidante might be the guy at the gym who, when you fell after trying to block a pass, not only helped you up, but asked, "Are you okay?" If he is asking if you are all right when you're hobbling off the court, he might also be someone you can talk to about whatever else is going on in your life. If you start telling your truth, the people who aren't meant to be there will fall away because they can't join in a conversation about your human revolution and evolution. And when you tell your story about how you finally glimpsed the real you, and how excited you were by what you saw, you'll be amazed at how many others will want to hear more, and even share their own journeys of self-discovery.

To be vulnerable is to be strong. To be open is to be free, and that freedom allows you to cast off the shadows that cloud your mirror.

Each of us has our own intricate journey. Only we know all the steps we took along the way, where we came from, who we came from. The hunter knows nothing about that, cares nothing for it, and he or she definitely has no right to dictate our stories.

So tell your own. Write it down. Share it with those who you believe you can trust. Then, you can become like the ancestors with their proverbs, offering guidance and an example to other Black boys and men about how to embrace and express their vulnerability as well.

Who are you really? That is the lifelong question our soul is asking, the reason for our finite trips around the sun. And when you find the answer, you can shatter that funhouse mirror and gaze upon a reflection that is truly your own.

WHAT TO TAKE AWAY

✳ **Finding the words.** What do you say to yourself about you? Who gave you those words? Say the answers to those questions out loud. Jot them in a journal. You may discover that you need to create and recite a new script about the real and authentic you.

✳ **Ask for directions.** Every single one of us feels lost at some point. Don't be afraid to ask for guidance. It's a sign of strength.

✳ **It doesn't always take a village.** Seek out a family member, teammate, or friend to share with. If you don't feel safe or heard, walk away. But don't stop looking, your person is waiting to hold your heart and story.

CHAPTER 4

The Only One in the Room

"When they approach me, they see only my surroundings, themselves, or figments of their imagination, indeed, everything and anything except me."

—RALPH ELLISON, *INVISIBLE MAN*

Dr. K's office sat across from Gramercy Park. It's a beautiful space, but unlike Central Park farther uptown, or Tompkins Square in the East Village, Gramercy was (and continues to be) basically off limits to anybody who didn't live in the pricey apartments around the park's edge. You literally had to have a key to open the gate and stroll inside.

One afternoon, I'd arrived early for my appointment, so I took a seat on the stoop of Dr. K's building. Dozens of men and women passed me, all of them white. No one looked me in the eye. They didn't even nod in my direction. It was as if I wasn't there.

I was still trying to climb out of the emotional pit my father's suicide had left me in. Now, looking at that locked gate across the street, watching all these white folks walk past like I was invisible, I felt empty, like I was nothing.

Finally, Dr. K arrived, and we went up to her office.

"I'm feeling really low today," I told her. "Like I'm a nobody."

She looked surprised. "What do you mean?" she asked. "You're a star on Broadway! You are on top of the world."

Then I explained to her how alone I'd felt sitting on that stoop, overlooked and locked out. I was a grown man, a professional who'd racked up a whole stack of accolades, and all those white folks simply refused to see me.

It's profoundly lonely to feel like you're cloaked in a fog. You can't see out, and no one even bothers trying to see in. If you were like my dad, believing there was no one to reach out to, I could understand how easy it would be to get to the end of your rope—the end of your hope—and give up.

Thankfully I had a mother who encouraged me to seek counseling, and I had people like Laura Linney and the masseuse, Gunilla, who led me to Dr. K. I felt comfortable talking to her about feeling invisible. I could talk to her about being deep in despair. And I was still sharing my dreams.

As I jotted down notes in my journals, I became aware of patterns. Sometimes I was in an attic or a basement, isolated, boxed in. But most often, I was on an athletic field, the arena where I'd spent so much time as a kid. Those dreams reflected whether I was on offense or defense in my life. If I felt I was dictating my experiences day to day, I'd dream that I was moving toward the goal line, while if I felt someone was trying to steer me in a direction that suited their own beliefs and agenda, I might dream I was the guard on the court, or that I was on the track running hurdles.

That was how I lived my life as a Black man. Overpreparing,

working extra hard, careful not to miss a step, and always alert to the vibe of others around me. It's why the older I got, the fewer tears I shed and the less vulnerable I became. I learned to live life on offense or defense because I was often the only Black boy in the room.

———————

I was born on March 12, 1960, and in the first years of my life, my family moved frequently. We went from Inkster, Michigan, where I could hear the trains whistle as I went to sleep, to Detroit, first to a building on Dundee Street and then to an apartment carved out of an old mansion on West Grand Boulevard, a few addresses down from Hitsville, Motown's original home. Then, in the spring of 1969, my parents bought their first house.

It was in a nearly all-white neighborhood in the northwest corner of the city. Although we and a couple other Black families were integrating the block, we didn't have to struggle through any *Raisin in the Sun*–type resistance. I guess our white neighbors didn't see any reason to get upset because they knew they'd be pulling up stakes and leaving before long.

Two years before we moved to Appoline Street, Detroit had gone up in flames. Folks set the city on fire after the police arrested dozens of Black men and women partying at an after-hours club known as a "blind pig." Then, a year later, it seemed like the embers had barely cooled when the world found out Martin Luther King Jr. had been assassinated.

Black people were fed up. Black people were angry. Dr. King's murder accelerated a sea change in how many saw the struggle for freedom and the best ways to get it. Black folks were pumping their fists, rocking twelve-inch Afros, and quoting Eldridge Cleaver. The words "Black Power" rang out everywhere. And when a former Tuskegee Airman named Coleman Young launched a campaign to become Detroit's first Black mayor and won, he carried that same activist spirit right into City Hall.

"We don't need y'all," was the message he sent to the city's white folks. "This is OUR city."

They didn't need to hear it twice. Believe me when I tell you that over the course of the summer of '69, it seemed like all the white people in Detroit simply vanished. It was like a *Twilight Zone* episode where you wake up in the morning and a whole community has disappeared. But this wasn't science fiction, and that sudden shift had a rippling, life-altering effect on everyone who fled and everyone who was left behind. Not just in Detroit, but in Cleveland, Newark, Compton, and so many other cities that experienced the same transition.

Cecilie and I didn't mind the change. Though we hadn't encountered any hostility when we moved to Appoline Street, being surrounded again by nothing but Black folks felt comfortable. But when the city's complexion changed, you could see the drop in resources almost immediately. There were more potholes that seemed to never get filled, more dilapidated buildings left to sag until they fell down. And then there was the diminishing quality of many of our local schools.

When our parents noticed that we were getting in more fights in the classroom and at recess, they plucked Cecilie and me out of our all-Black schools right in the middle of the semester and sent us to small, virtually all-white Catholic academies across town.

I can only imagine the conversation that led to that decision. For many of the folks in my parents' generation, a good factory job and a small house were their American dream. Their aspirations for themselves and even their children were narrow because of how much they'd already overcome just to make the journey from Mississippi and Alabama to carve out a less tenuous life in the North. Many believed finishing high school, getting a job, and starting a family were more than good enough. But that was not the dream my parents had for my sister and me.

Mommy and Daddy bought a house in a mostly white neighborhood thinking they'd see their property value go up and up and up, and now they were essentially back in a segregated community, having to pay for Catholic school to make sure their kids got a good education. Our parents didn't ask if we wanted to make the switch. They didn't even sit us down to tell us about the move. Cecilie and I found out we were transferring schools the next morning.

We must have imagined we'd be going to some boarding school far away or maybe selling the house. I can't recall what went through the minds of our eight- and ten-year-old selves, but we literally packed our little suitcases and sat them by the door.

The next morning, we saw that our suitcases were back in the closet. But instead of walking to school, my mother's friend Claire Michaud picked us up and drove us to Mother of Our Savior, our new school across town. That commute would be our daily routine for the next five years.

Mommy and Daddy never offered an explanation, and we knew better than to ask questions. They were our parents. They made the rules. And there definitely wasn't any discussion about how to navigate this new all-white world where we suddenly had to stand when a teacher entered the room and recite the rosary twice a day. There was no offer of therapy to talk to us about how we felt. We just had to figure it all out.

It was like that for Black children all over the country in the 1960s and early 1970s, I'd imagine. After the U.S. Supreme

Court's decision in *Brown v. Board of Education of Topeka* that declared segregation unconstitutional, it took several years for the law to be broadly enforced. But gradually more and more Black boys and girls began integrating public and private schools, and their parents didn't know a thing about what their children would experience. They just sent them out the door every morning with their book bags and a prayer, hoping for the best.

On the other side of that transition were the white teachers, administrators, and students. Even if they weren't spitting and screaming like a lot of those hideously racist folks in the news clips filmed down South, nobody was asking the new Black kids how they were doing or what they could do to help. At least I don't remember any priest or teacher at Mother of Our Savior checking to see if I was struggling to fit in.

It got to be confusing traveling between the neighborhood where the faces resembled my own, and a school where I was surrounded by all white children. I basically had to become bilingual, careful I didn't use the "wrong" voice in the "wrong" place. I didn't want to slip into Black slang in the schoolyard or reveal that I secretly dug the Rolling Stones as much as I did James Brown when I was at my best friend's house next door.

Still, sometimes I slipped.

"Daaaang, Court," my buddy Jimmy said one day, his eyes wide and incredulous. "You sound like a white boy!"

I'm sure there were thousands of Black boys like me being told they "talked white" back home while being looked down on if they carelessly let an "ain't" fly by in class. We Black boys who were suddenly the only ones in the room, integrating new environments, felt like outsiders wherever we were. But we didn't know how to discuss what we were going through, not even with each other.

Maybe we were scared that if we acknowledged this tightrope we were straddling, we'd lose our balance and tumble to the ground. When we crashed, we'd dash our parents' dreams, and maybe our own as well.

I didn't even discuss what was happening with my sister. Each of us just adjusted on our own. I learned to shift my cadence to fit my environment, becoming an actor years before I had an actual career on the stage. Other times I felt like myself, though I was revealing only a small piece of me, because, like all of us, I was many things—the studious boy who loved Peter Frampton LIVE! and the kid who carried an Afro pick with a fist etched in the handle. I was the fan who appreciated The Beatles and the young man who could break out and do a mean James Brown strut at the drop of a needle.

It was becoming clear that my trajectory was changing. My path was veering in a vastly different direction from that of my buddy Greg, who lived around the corner and would end up dead at the age of sixteen, and my best friend Darren, who got married and started working for the gas company right after high school. I'd always appreciate that well of blackness I'd been immersed in, but I was stretching beyond my all-Black cocoon.

The first stop on the journey into my future was that nearly all-white block in Northwest Detroit. The next was Mother of Our Savior, the school I attended from fourth to sixth grade. Then it was on to middle school at St. Mary's of Redford.

And then there was the Boys' Club of Highland Park (girls weren't admitted until decades later), which truly put me at the crossroads.

The Boys & Girls Clubs of America are a national network of 5000 clubs that have been building children up for more than 160 years, teaching them life skills and providing them with mentorship and support. I was maybe in the third grade when my parents began taking me to the Highland Park club after school to make sure I didn't get into any trouble out in the street. Soon I was spending my Saturdays there as well.

Though all the kids were Black, the staff and administrators were nearly all white, including Mr. George Browne, who was our summer camp counselor. We absolutely loved him. One of his favorite sayings was, "Your soul may belong to the world, but your ass belongs to me." It was the kind of thing our fathers or uncles would have said. He was one of us.

"Did you hear what Big G said today?" we'd whisper to each other as we cracked up laughing.

When I was eight years old, I attended the summer day camp for the first time, and sometimes we'd head to a nearby campground and do a sleepover. We'd sing songs, play kick the can, and stay up till dawn in our bunk beds, joking around. I'm sure if I went back to that camp today, fifty years later, I'd find some ramshackle cabins and a worn-out dining hall. But in my memory, it was an oasis.

Mr. Browne would make us pancakes in the morning and help us slap together Sloppy Joes and s'mores over a campfire at night. I went every summer until I was thirteen, and as I got older, Mr. Browne made me a junior counselor who helped supervise the younger boys.

With all the time I spent at the club, Mr. Browne and my father also became very close. They were similar in many ways, hardworking guys who didn't take any nonsense off kids but who were ultimately more admired than feared. One day Mr. Browne told my dad about a school in Beverly Hills, Michigan. It was called Detroit Country Day School.

Mr. Browne thought I had a good chance of being accepted, and there were scholarships available if we needed help with the tuition, which was three thousand dollars a year. That was a small fortune in the 1970s, when the average in-state tuition to attend a public university was roughly $500 a year, or less. I remember the day my parents and I finally visited the campus. For a boy from the inner city, it was like going to Shangri-La. The gym even had a glass backboard. I'd never seen anything like that on the playground back home. "This," I thought, "is where I want to be."

Still, even though I applied in the seventh grade and passed the entrance exam, I didn't get in. I was disappointed, but since I didn't really know all I might be missing, I didn't mope for long. There was too much fun happening back in my all-Black world.

There was a park near us, and during the freezing Michigan winters, a sheet of ice formed on the lawn that was thick enough for ice skating. Then, the city built an indoor hockey rink about a half mile away and that became the spot. I got a pair of skates for Christmas, and every Saturday night I'd join all these beautiful Black folks gliding around the ice.

There were many boys in particular who were spectacular skaters. They weren't doing figure eights and curly cues. They whipped around the rink like lightning, fast, and clean and sharp enough I believed to be able to hang on any professional hockey team.

One older guy named Leo would often take the lead, and the rest of us, not nearly as graceful but trying our best, would follow behind like he was the Pied Piper.

"Daddy, I want to play ice hockey," I told my dad one night, breathless and shivering and happy.

"Courtney," he said, shaking his head. "You ain't playing no hockey."

Maybe he imagined me getting chased around by some burly

Canadian players who figured hockey was *their* sport. Perhaps he imagined me getting slammed with a puck and ending up with no teeth. Perhaps he didn't want to pay that money for ice time and equipment. Or maybe he just didn't want to wake up at 3:30 in the morning to get me to the rink. Whatever the reason, hockey was out.

But a different dream of mine was about to come true.

———

The next time I took the test for Country Day, I was accepted and invited to start attending in the ninth grade.

I still wanted to go, but I was getting older and gaining a better understanding of things like work, and money and sacrifice. I realized that this school with the rolling green lawns and sparkling gym had to be really expensive. I thought it had to be hard enough on my parents to send my sister and me to Catholic school. Country Day was probably out of reach.

Cecilie was going to Cass Tech, the best public high school in the city. I figured I'd stay at St. Mary's of Redford and go on to high school at Cass until one weekend, when I was doing some chores in the basement and Dad called me over.

"Son," he said, "where do you want to go to high school?"

"Well," I said a bit hesitantly. "Country Day. But we can't afford it."

"No, Son," he said. "Your mother and I talked about it, and if that's where you want to go, we're going to do what we need to do to send you there."

Just like that, my life shifted.

From my first day officially on campus, I loved everything about Country Day. It was just the newness of it, how the waxy floors literally glistened, and all the male students had to wear ties. I didn't know why so many of the other kids, many of whom had been there for years, weren't as excited as I was. I wanted to play every sport, to join every club.

In our class of sixty-four students, maybe ten of us were Black. After years in Catholic school, I'd gotten used to being the only, or one of the few, Black kids in class. And my study habits were solid so I was confident I could make the grades that would draw everybody's admiration. Still, I didn't know anybody. And I wasn't just in school with a bunch of strangers; I was attending classes with the scions of Michigan's wealthiest families.

On top of all that, I was traveling so far to campus every day, I couldn't hang with the people back on my block like I did before. The distance between us grew greater. I was truly in between worlds.

But Country Day quickly welcomed me.

Not long after the school year started, someone approached me about doing announcements for the school. I said yes and started taking over the PA system in the morning to announce the winners of a tennis match, the details of the morning assembly, and other daily events. I really struggled in the beginning though to pronounce some of my classmates' names.

Bar-tho-lomewwwwu Gonsalvez.

Zenyuhhh Mulholland.

All my stumbling made for a daily comedy show. But the faculty was patient, and everyone in school got to know me. I was even on the seniors' radar.

I also had another way to fit in—sports. Athletics had always been the space that earned me acceptance, even back when I was playing football at St. Mary's, tackling, scoring, and quarterbacking in the seventh and eighth grades.

Today, as I seek to connect with other Black men about their emotional struggles and challenges, I realize that life might have been harder for some of the other Black students at Country Day who didn't have athletics to ease their way. When I arrived there in the fall of 1974, the school had only been integrated for a few years and it had also only recently begun admitting young ladies.

My classmates and I were in the vanguard as Country Day began to awkwardly grapple with a change the entire nation was undergoing, fitfully trying to become the equitable place it had never been. And there were no resources provided, no discussions, only silence.

I didn't have much time, though, to observe my classmates' struggles or to reflect on all the changes we were going through. Because we couldn't afford the private school bus service, my parents paid an upper classman, Brian Miller, to take me to school every morning. Then after practice, Michael Young, a senior on the basketball, football, and track teams, would drive me home. When I wasn't working out, I was in some little cubbyhole doing homework. On Saturdays I had games, and Sundays I was studying.

I was busy achieving. I was busy being accepted. And I had sports to help usher me through—until the day I found out how some of the people I believed were in my corner really saw me.

It happened during my senior year, but the experience that helped me know how to deal with that moment had occurred years earlier.

When I was in the seventh grade, I began to have a problem with my right knee. A big lump had suddenly formed, and I was diagnosed with Osgood-Schlatter disease. The doctor said I would have to give up football, at least temporarily, and I was devastated. I loved the game. But my parents explained the situation to me well.

"You can play now," they said, "or you can play later. You

take care of yourself, and do what you need to do, or you keep playing and kiss high school football goodbye."

They were telling me I had to be patient in order to heal. It was the hardest thing in the world to be twelve years old and still wrap my knee with Ace bandages every morning and walk stiffly like an old man for six months. But learning to delay my gratification, to wait for what I wanted, proved to be a defining moment in my life.

I didn't know it then, but that was the first time I had to let the mud settle and the water clear. It was a lesson I would need to remember and reclaim years later after my father killed himself. And it was a lesson that guided me my last year of high school, when I learned what it was to be reduced to nothing more than a Black athlete, someone who was supposed to be grateful and do what I was told.

I planned to take a break from the basketball team that winter. We'd lost our beloved coach, who'd gone to another school, and frankly, I was exhausted from playing three sports for four years. I wanted to rest up for track season and focus on my college applications. One day when I was in the library, someone from the office came to find me. The headmaster wanted to see me in his office.

I wasn't worried. I hadn't done anything wrong. When I got there, he and I went back and forth with some small talk. Then he let me know why I was there.

"I hear you're not playing basketball this season," he said.

"Yeah," I said, explaining how I wanted to focus on college admissions and track instead.

He sat back.

"Well, we kind of want you to play," he said.

I didn't know whether to be flattered or concerned. "I know," I said finally. "But I'm burnt out."

"We *realllly* want you to play," he repeated.

I was getting antsy. "Okay. I told you I don't want to play. So what are you saying?"

"If you don't play, we'll revoke your athletic scholarship."

Scholarship? I wasn't on an athletic scholarship. I'd played all these years because I wanted to, because I was literally a team player. I'd done announcements, mentored students, and gotten straight A's. I'd worked my tail off, and now I was tired. Yet here was this arrogant man threatening to kick me out of school.

It was a racist move. But I understood.

He wanted to put me in my place. I was a Black kid who didn't come from money. I wasn't on an athletic scholarship, but in his mind, I should have been. I owed them.

I'd floated into that office feeling good but walked out in a state of shock. When I got home and told my parents what happened, they were furious. They even talked about suing. But I'd made a decision.

"Forget it," I said. "I'm going to play."

They said I didn't have to, but I'd made up my mind. I had to deal with something uncomfortable now, so I could play later. So I could graduate, and soar and achieve all the great things that were supposed to come from this experience.

I was captain of the team that season, and as I'd predicted, we were absolutely terrible. We were particularly awful on offense. But off the court, living as a young Black man in America, I knew how to grab the ball and score, how to not only survive, but thrive. I lived much of my life on offense. That's why I'd decided to play.

———

At the end of the school year, there was an assembly for the seniors and their families. I'd already gotten what I thought was the sweetest award, acceptance to Harvard, and I didn't expect to get any special honors. But my teachers said that it was important for my parents to be there, so Mommy and Daddy took the day off from work and came.

After announcing the valedictorian and athletic MVP, it was time for the presentation of the Headmaster's Cup. It was the highest accolade Country Day had to offer, given to the student who most embodied the school's ideals of mind, body, and spirit.

"And the recipient of the Headmaster's Cup is... Courtney B. Vance!"

The audience stood up and roared! As I approached the stage, I looked back at my dad fumbling for his glasses, tears streaming down his face. It may have been the only time I ever saw him cry.

My decision to go ahead and play despite the ugly threat that led me to do it is probably what clinched that honor for me. That cup represented all that I'd learned from cobbling together my short life's lessons and figuring out a game plan of my own.

Still, I wish I'd had someone to lean on as I gained my footing, that I'd known I didn't have to keep my confusing duality to myself. I had some Black classmates who struggled later in their marriages and careers. They'd picked up a bunch of business contacts and a pack of credentials, but also accumulated a whole lot of trauma being the only one or one of a few in cold, colorless spaces.

Maybe if a teacher, a coach, or a neighborhood elder had told them they understood how hard it must be straddling two worlds, those classmates would have become healthy enough to achieve all that they yearned for. Maybe if I'd let them know that, despite my popularity, I'd had moments when I felt bewildered and alone too, they would have realized stumbling along was as human and worthy of acknowledgment as so-called success.

For too long, Black people have felt the need to prove we're worthy of citizenship, of acceptance, and we've often had no road map as we went along. And fearful that we were the only ones struggling, we didn't feel we could share the mental pressures of all that injustice.

When my own children had similar challenges decades later, adjusting to a new school, meeting heightened expectations, I let them know that I had gone through the same turmoil, and no, they didn't have to figure it out by themselves.

Suicide and silence have taught me the role that I can play. A need for solace and healing has taught me the bridge that I can be. I've learned a lot of lessons. And I'm passing them on.

All by Myself

For Black men, being the only one in the room is, well, complicated.

On the one hand, it can be isolating and frightening to have all eyes on you. But depending on the room and the circumstances, you could also experience the illusion, or the actual experience, of being deemed special, not only by those in the room but by the folks on the outside looking in.

Yet the spotlight is like a pendulum, swinging back and forth, and the blade cuts both ways.

What does it mean to be both objectified and celebrated? When you are seemingly welcomed into white spaces, particularly bastions of white privilege, you can begin to believe you really are better.

But what if you are stripped of whatever got you the ticket to the club? What if, like Courtney, you no longer want to play ball? What if you are a corporate climber who, after witnessing others experiencing discrimination, decides to speak up and no longer stay quiet? When you step out of line, or when you enter an environment where people don't know you and reduce you to the same stereotypes that shadow so many of your brothers, that's when the emotional whiplash comes.

I've done a lot of work with professional athletes and entertainers, and I've spoken to them about what it feels like to have people jumping up and down in a stadium chanting their name while also knowing that if they were to take off their uniforms and put on a cap that hid their face, those same fans might react to them with hostility or fear.

Many chose to tuck that understanding into their subconscious because it was too painful to sit and contemplate. Like the anger Courtney felt when he was called into the headmaster's office, it can be galling to realize that the folks in the bleachers, the school principal standing on the sidelines, or the colleague you occasionally have drinks with want you around only when you are making them feel good, pulling in the big accounts, or providing them entertainment. They don't want you, however, to date their daughters. They don't want you to sit at their dinner table or to move in next door. Or maybe they wouldn't mind, as long as you are the only one. I have been the only one invited for a sleepover by a white friend, who the next morning uninvited me to Sunday School, "because her church might be uncomfortable, and not understand." It's painful to be dismissed or isolated as the only one.

DO YOU SEE ME?

Black men also live with the contradiction of being highly scrutinized and invisible at the same time. They know that whenever they are in non-Black spaces, they are being watched, sometimes with admiration, sometimes with envy, often with fear. Courtney has spent a lifetime in the most homogeneous of spaces—prep schools; the Ivy League; the theater, which is literally the Great White Way; and finally Hollywood. He has achieved in all of them, reaping accolades, awards, and applause.

And yet there was that day when he went to his counseling session, and he dealt with the incongruity of being seen by Dr. K and not seen by all the people who walked by. How do you hold those two realities? That paradox is one of the reasons so many Black men feel alienated. And it is also why, though you may have flashes of recognition like Courtney did that afternoon, you choose much of the time not to face it.

Black men who are achieving, getting elected president of the PTA, promoted to the C-suite, or making it happen in Hollywood often have a whole internal script to reassure themselves that they are not bothered by such contradictions. They tell themselves that they don't resent that their white peers don't have to deal with such a duality. They try to believe that it's not painful or messy to know deep down that their special status is fragile and can be quickly taken away, or that if they are considered special, it means so many who look like them are not. They live in denial.

But all denial is not the same. Conscious denial can be necessary for wellness. Unconscious denial can be downright dangerous.

When you know what's going on, yet shut off that awareness from time to time, that can preserve your mental health and help you to achieve a greater purpose. Sometimes you need to see the whole story, and other times you need to let some of that narrative fade into the background.

For instance, if you're getting a chance to run a department that generates millions of dollars in revenue but has very little diversity, you can immediately ask those who've promoted you, "Why am I the only Black man here?" Or you can take the position, resolve to bring about change once you have the power, and save those questions for another day. You bring the knowledge you need at the time to the table and leave behind what won't work for you in the moment.

That kind of conscious denial is very different from checking out completely, never acknowledging all the paradoxes that circumscribe your life.

Let me say here, that unconscious denial is also a coping mechanism, a way to mentally survive when those absurd inconsistencies are more than you can bear. The problem is that what lives in the unconscious doesn't stay buried. When it bursts into the open, it may erupt in depression, bitterness, or rage. That emotional explosion may culminate in addiction, violence, or suicide. The refusal to recognize and reconcile their conflicting realities is why so many Black men self-destruct or wander through their lives not understanding why they might not be able to stay faithful, keep a job, or sleep through the night.

As hard as it may be to look at the roots of your trauma, having that kind of insight is powerful even if sometimes you have to knowingly look away. Becoming whole literally means bringing your whole story into your consciousness, even if sometimes you need to shift it to the back of your mind to attain a goal, to avoid a pitfall, or just to make it to the next morning.

AN ORDINARY GUY

And what if you are not the exceptional man in the room? What if you are the Black boy who will never lead an organization, the man who isn't on the C-level track, the ordinary guy who is never treated like he is "special" or unique?

Even Black men at the heights of their professions sometimes struggle with "imposter syndrome," feeling that they are not good enough, that luck, and not hard work, has gotten them where they are and that the rug can be pulled from beneath them at any moment. The average everyday man has even more challenges to overcome.

For white men, systemic racism and patriarchy grandfathers them into the security that they don't have to be a superstar to have value. He can simply be a good dad, or a hard worker, and he is deemed worthy and above men from other racial backgrounds. But for Black men, there's a different kind of pressure, a weight that comes from knowing, even unconsciously, that you were once viewed as a fraction of a human being, and oftentimes have been treated as even less than that.

For those Black men who aren't necessarily the top students, the fraternity leaders, or the board members, they often don't have the same psychological cushion as their brothers who are singled out and celebrated. It can be even more difficult to see themselves as valuable in a culture that sees them as expendable. They feel dismissed and forgotten. And such emotions can be a breeding ground for many ills, from the physical to the financial, to the spiritual and emotional.

Loneliness and isolation also smother creativity. A Black man existing in a prison of solitude is less likely to imagine his future, or to cultivate and nurture his dreams. He may be going through the motions, working long hours, paying his bills, but if you looked into his eyes, you'd see that there was no one home. He cannot figure out all he is capable of, and so, too often, neither can those who surround and love him.

Talking trash on the corner with his boys or over drinks after work doesn't usually lead to an airing of his true frustrations. Indeed, the chatter about sex, partying all weekend, or a financial achievement may mask his hurt, enabling him to ignore or sidestep the raw feelings he has about other chapters of his life. Whether he faces them or not, one way or another, the inability to voice his truth or envision his future will begin to wear him down.

And then, on top of the ordinary daily challenges we all deal with—trying to juggle work and home, trying to manage relationships and extinguish life's constant small fires—there is the ever-present backdrop of racial discrimination. Racism is exhausting. It is also unavoidable. Trying to navigate it in isolation is very different than navigating it as a tribe. But unfortunately, too many Black men are doing it solo.

THE BIG LIE

It is interesting that Courtney often dreamed of himself being on offense. The rule following and overpreparing that have largely defined his overachieving life is in line with the more common posture Black men take on—and that is being on defense.

Relatively few Black men feel they are staying ahead of the hunter. Even on offense, the bottom line is to defend himself against racism. It's to stand up against systemic, bigoted power. It's to beat back the big lie.

In the aftermath of the 2020 presidential election, Donald Trump and his political party and supporters went on a relentless campaign to claim he'd won a race against President Joe Biden that Trump actually lost by more than seven million popular votes and seventy-four votes in the electoral college.

It's been rightly dubbed the "Big Lie." But there is a bigger lie that sits at its foundation, and that is the lie of white supremacy, a fiction that fuels inequities in this society in areas ranging from housing, to education, to criminal justice. It also leads to imposter syndrome, the idea held by some Black men who've penetrated white spaces that they don't deserve to be there.

Black men are not the imposters. It is the supposed meritocracy that governs the environments they're in that is fraudulent.

And then there are those Black men who don't get a chance to be in those spaces in the first place. For those who don't have the grades or the financial resources to get into the top-ranked schools, who don't have jobs that earn them six figures, or the ability to not just survive but thrive, it's not that their brains weren't as good, or that their skills weren't as sharp as those who are said to have made it. It's the web of systems, built over four hundred years and designed to make them believe they can't handle the tasks at hand, that conspire to lock them out.

It's important to note that penetrating exclusive white spaces should not be the marker of success. Black communities and institutions are just as worthy, and being able to feed your intellectual curiosity and tap into your talents within them can be even more gratifying. Being the only or one of the few in white environments can also be alienating and distressing.

But for those who've wanted certain opportunities and been denied, when you realize it was the access that was deficient, and not you, you can see roads not taken in a completely different light. And you recognize another truth. The others in the room who seem so confident that they belong are not any more competent than you. Indeed, they may be less fit, and often they are less resilient because they had so much less to overcome to get where they are, and so much less to navigate in order to stay.

It is important for Black boys and men to be reminded, and to realize, that they are more than capable. That they deserve to be in the room in multitudes. It is the system that is the imposter.

WAKE UP AND SHOW UP

So how do you accept the paradox? How do you deal with a system designed to squash your dreams? How do you face the unbearable?

Slowly and gently.

As Black boys and men ask themselves "Who Am I?" there may be the painful realization that society refuses to see them for who they truly are. They are watched, stereotyped, and labeled while their complexity and full humanity are ignored.

It is difficult, as you are waking up to your full potential, and showing up for the man staring back at you from the mirror, to face that you must still battle outsiders and systems that want to keep you stunted or in a box. They don't want you emotionally healthy because that makes you harder to manipulate, and harder to control. That self-awareness makes you even more questioning of institutions that send Black men to jail for voting and give a slap on the wrist to white men who foment and engage in an insurrection.

That's why there will definitely come a time, as you explore how you came to be who you are and grapple with the impact of your experiences, that you cannot do that excavation alone. You will need to connect and share your story with others.

You are unrolling a rich tapestry. Where do I hurt? Who am I really? Why do others refuse to see me as I do? Why is my very existence a threat?

As you navigate your inner world, you will sometimes need others who can keep you from going in circles. As you tell your truth, you need others to bear witness, to affirm your right to move through whatever you are feeling, and to simply hold you up if you fear that, if you dig any deeper, you will lose your mind.

Without support, it is easy to bury whatever thoughts and feelings rise to the surface. And then you risk an eventual emotional rupture that can keep you from having the relationships, the achievements, or the peace of mind that you deserve. Burying your feelings and living in isolation can eventually catch up with the best of you, making you physically, emotionally, and spiritually sick.

A therapist can provide that safe space where you can do that emotional exploration. But not everyone is able to access counseling, or comfortable with the idea of going to a mental health professional. Others may have a good friend they can talk to, but some will find their inner circle is just not able or willing to bear their pain.

Fortunately, there are other resources rising up to offer Black men and boys support.

Black men and women are increasingly creating safe spaces where their brothers can gather. Jay Barnett, a former professional football player who sought counseling after trying to take his life by suicide twice, is now a highly sought-after mental health coach. In 2022, he partnered with Hope Allen, creator and producer of the Just Heal Bro Tour to invite Black men in communities across the United States to come together to speak about their emotional health.

"Our Black boys and now our Black men have not been given the opportunity to emote properly and healthily, so they've developed these negative coping skills and destructive habits," says Barnett, a key headliner for the tour, which is named for a book he wrote about his own mental health journey. "As long as people will allow us to create the space with the Just Heal Bro Tour, I'm going to keep showing up for them because somebody showed up for me."

Authenticity is key. There have been many initiatives put in place by government officials, including the Obama administration's "My Brother's Keeper," but despite their funding and fanfare, mental health indicators for Black boys and men have gotten worse, not better. Those efforts may have been launched with the best of intentions, but for Black boys and men, so isolated and alienated, so misled and mistreated, there's a level of intimacy that is often necessary for emotional repair to begin.

If there is trauma happening on the street corner, treatment can also happen there as well. A young man who gets the support he needs to undergo a personal transformation can take what he's learned back to his boys, and also his family. He can let them know that there's a different way to move, a different way to be. Black men can offer and receive support where they are most comfortable, whether it's a neighborhood park, the aisle of a grocery store, or in a barber's chair.

Dr. Howard Stevenson, a professor at the University of Pennsylvania and renowned psychologist who specializes in healing from racial trauma, has actually trained barbers to clinically engage with their clients. In the Black community, barbers have long done healing work, soothing and touching those who sit in their booths, allowing them to vent or to just have a moment of pampering and rest. So Dr. Stevenson has spent decades helping them lean into the crucial therapeutic roles that they play.

It might go like this: Instead of asking a client whose wife is sick how she's doing, a barber can go deeper: *How is she, and how are you taking care of yourself as you tend to her and cope with the fear of what could happen?* He can refer his patron to an acquaintance who's gone through something similar, or maybe hand him the contact information for a support group that is helping others grapple with a similar situation.

When a young man sitting in the barber's chair is asked how he is really doing, when he offers him a phone number to a group where he can safely engage in fellowship, or just grants him a little time to talk and breathe, that man can walk out of that shop not only with a sharp fade, but with the realization that he is not alone. That may be just the remedy he needs, and the push that will motivate him to seek even more support.

When we enable Black men to talk through their trauma, we give them the room to recall who they have always been, or to claim their power to begin again. We shore up their strength to pursue their dreams, to be big, and Black and bold.

Then they won't need anyone else to tell them they are enough. Give Black men and boys the time and space where they can put down their burdens and see their true reflections, and they'll be more than able to tell themselves.

WHAT TO TAKE AWAY

* **Denial can serve a purpose.** But facing challenges is vital so your emotions don't erupt in unhealthy ways.
* **Don't assume.** Often we feel that we are the only ones struggling, but when one reveals their trials, it encourages others to detail theirs as well. You may be the only Black boy or man in certain settings, but don't assume you are the only person who feels isolated, insecure, anxious or depressed.
* **Carving out authentic spaces.** Just Heal, Bro, The Confess Project, Moms of Black Boys United, and other initiatives are increasing as Black men and women create places where Black boys and men can gather to share their stories and receive mental health and wellness support.
* **Therapy and healing can occur wherever a Black man stands or sits.** Not everyone can or wants to see a professional counselor. But therapeutic support can be found in nontraditional spaces, including a barber's chair.

CHAPTER 5

Suffer the Little Children

"I have such thoughts, I have such strange thoughts."

—WILLY LOMAN, *DEATH OF A SALESMAN*

Sometimes those around you can do everything right. They ask you where does it hurt? They ask how can they help? They draw you close. They raise you up. And still, it isn't enough.

I met Bobby Robinson through mutual friends more than a decade ago. We hit it off, stayed in touch, and grew to be close friends. So close that he and his wife, Patricia, asked Angela and me to be godparents to their children.

My godson was maybe twelve years old, and his sister was eleven. They were beautiful kids, curious, kind, and well-mannered. Well, at least most of the time.

One weekend when we were over at Bobby and Patricia's house, I went to get a glass from the kitchen, and while walking back to the den, I spotted Patricia and my godson in the hallway.

"Give me your hand," Patricia said.

"Ooooh," I thought, remembering when my mother spoke to me in that same tone when I was a little boy. I didn't know what my godson had done, but I knew he was in trouble.

"I didn't *do* anything," he pleaded.

"Give. Me. Your. Hand," Patricia said.

He reluctantly lifted his palm. Patricia gave it a tiny whack with her comb.

That's the way she and Bobby did it. They didn't tolerate any nonsense, and if their kids stepped out of line, they were disciplined. But most of the time the Robinsons were hugging, praising, and showering their two amazing children with love. Angela and I were in our forties when we had our babies, and we were always looking for role models, folks we felt were parenting successfully. Bobby and Patricia were two we admired from afar.

We spent hours and hours together, and the Robinson kids became like an older brother and sister to our son, Slater, and our daughter, Bronwyn. Angela and I loved our godchildren fiercely.

But no matter how close you are to someone, you don't know everything that's going on in their home. Nor should you. People have a right to decide what they want to share, and if and when they want to share it. So I didn't learn until much later that my godson began to struggle emotionally when he went off to college.

That's not uncommon. I remember my first semester at Harvard. I was miserable living away from home for the first time, and I really missed Michigan. Then, during one of our school vacations, the young lady I'd been dating since high school told me she might want to break up. She was attending Swarthmore in Pennsylvania and wasn't fully comfortable with our long-distance romance. I told her we could make it work and went back to Cambridge cautiously hopeful I'd changed her mind. But the "Dear Courtney" letter was waiting for me as soon as I got back to my dorm. I was devastated.

My godson, who was a talented musician and a member of the

college band, suffered a similar heartbreak. He was also struggling with a chemical imbalance that made an emotional setback like that even harder to recover from. To everyone looking in, he was a smart, handsome kid who was also a great drummer, but he was spiraling. Finally, his parents decided to bring him home.

That seemed to be what he needed, to be with those who loved him most, to be in a safe place where he could get his bearings. He began tutoring some of the kids his dad coached on a local pee wee football team and was adjusting well. Everybody thought he was happy.

Then COVID-19 hit. The pandemic created a new challenge for so many young people, stripping away school, preventing them from socializing with their friends. They were isolated, and perhaps encountering death and serious illness for the first time. It also meant that if your child wasn't well, they might have to interact with a doctor by themselves as social distancing protocols prevented their loved ones from accompanying them into a medical office or hospital.

That's what happened with my godson. Twice, after he experienced a mental health episode, Bobby and Patricia took him to the hospital—but they had to wait outside in their car while he went in alone.

You know young people. You ask them how they're doing, and they mumble, "Okay," or "Fine." They might not have the language to express what they're going through. Or they might understand how they're feeling but be too embarrassed to admit it.

"I'm good," he told the doctors. So they told him to continue with his therapy and sent him home.

Bobby and Patricia were dumbfounded. Yes, their son was calm now, but he could be hours or even minutes away from another emotional episode, trashing his room in frustration or crying uncontrollably. Then what were they going to do? They felt he needed medication. But the doctors didn't prescribe any.

They were right there at the hospital, twice, and they couldn't go in and advocate for their child or get any guidance on what to do. He was technically an adult, but still in need of support. Should they watch him twenty-four hours a day? Were they supposed to sleep beside him at night, like they did when he was a baby in his crib? They would have done all of that if a doctor they trusted only said so.

In between those harrowing episodes, my godson continued to be a wonderful big brother, and he kept working with the boys on his father's football team. He was trying to hold on. His loved ones were trying to keep him close. But they couldn't pull him out of his final spiral.

One day in 2020, on a date I don't want to remember, he hung himself in his room.

Having lived through my father's suicide didn't make my godson's death any less devastating. In some ways, it may have been even more traumatic, because the family had tried so hard to save him, and because he was so young with so much promise and possibility hovering on the horizon.

He was the Robinsons' baby boy, their older child, their only son. He was his sister's and Slater's and Bronwyn's big brother. For twenty-three years, the Robinsons had been a quartet, their lives filled with this beloved young man's rhythm, and now he was gone.

Though I wasn't really aware of it when I was younger, my sister, Cecilie, was also diagnosed with a chemical imbalance, and she'd been taking medication to stabilize her mood for decades. Our family saw no shame in her needing medicine.

Over time, it had become crystal clear that, along with therapy, those pills probably saved my sister's life.

Bobby and his wife believed their son should have been on medication. He didn't get it, and it cost them everything. My godson needed some damn medicine. And the system failed him.

The Robinsons aren't an anomaly. Our country's health care system is in shambles. Every one of us should have health insurance. Every one of us should have a doctor we can trust. But many folks still don't have coverage, and too many can't afford the copayments and deductibles even if they do. It's also a struggle to form a real relationship with a doctor. Folks are shuttled in and out of medical offices like cogs moving along an assembly line.

Bobby and Patricia didn't have the kind of connection with a family physician that made them feel comfortable calling and talking about whatever was going on with their son. And whoever was treating him either didn't care or wasn't perceptive enough to recognize what he needed. COVID made it hard for people to have an advocate with them in a hospital emergency room or a doctor's office, which is a terrible thing because it's important to have someone with us when we can't or don't know how to speak up for ourselves—when we don't know the questions to ask, or are too intimidated or out of sorts to ask them.

COVID created a crack in time, and how many people suffered during that moment? How many other parents or young people in distress couldn't get the help they needed? Who's going to pay for a life lost because the medical system didn't respond in the right way?

In the midst of their overwhelming heartache, the Robinsons suffered even more. Bobby, who worked in sales, was downsized.

Patricia was in a car accident. Yvette was in school, just trying to focus on her studies and weather the storm.

The Robinsons were enveloped by a loving community, but that's not always the case when a loved one dies. Sometimes people in your life disappear, not because they don't love you, but because grief brings up so many things inside folks that they just can't handle. Your loss unleashes their own memories or trauma, so they don't reach out because it's too much.

Death by suicide brings up another layer of emotions that may push people away. When someone passes from cancer, gets killed in a car accident, or finally loses their battle with diabetes, it's devastating but people understand. Suicide, however, still too often carries a stigma. People may feel that something was wrong with that person who killed themselves and maybe even something wrong with the family they left behind.

How could they do something like that?

Don't they know that's a sin?

Life is so precious, and they decided to just throw theirs away?

For those whose loved one takes their own life, the ostracization, the questions, just add to their devastation. That may make even some of those who survive want to take themselves out the same way.

The Robinsons were a God-fearing family and so they leaned on faith. And Angela and I joined the rest of their village, hugging them through their tears, kneeling down with them in prayer, and just supporting them in any way we could.

But I knew I had to do more.

Thirty years earlier, my father had killed himself. Now, my twenty-three-year-old godson had done the same thing. Two people I'd loved more than anyone in this world had taken their own lives. I thought, I can't do this again. I can't do this anymore. I've got to speak up. I've got to say something. We were losing too many people who couldn't find the hope to hang on.

There are so many young men like my godson, who seem to have everything to live for but can't get through a terribly bleak moment, who feel they can't bear to be in this life for one minute more. One suicide would be too many, but now it feels like an epidemic is coursing through the Black community like another plague and pandemic.

I understand that it's a point any of us could descend to. Without a foundation up under you, or a bridge to bring you back, getting to the other side of a situation that breaks your spirit or your heart can feel impossible. It's easy to forget, if you ever knew, what Psalm 30:5 tells us: "Weeping may endure for a night, but joy cometh in the morning."

I knew I needed to let my brothers, those who are young like my godson, and those in their senior years like my father was, know that it was okay to need therapy or medication to help them make it through. I needed to talk to them about how there were boys and men like themselves who were taking their own lives, and there was help out there, so they didn't have to take the same devastating and permanent step.

I knew we had to bring mental anguish and illness out of the shadows, to stop yelling "You crazy," like it's an insult. Because we all struggle, we all spiral, we all have moments when we are confused. So, by that definition, we're all crazy. The insults needed to stop. And the understanding needed to begin.

———

My godson's generation is dealing with forces and pressures that I could not have imagined when I was a kid. I grew up at a time when you got your music on vinyl, you had to wait seven days for a check to clear, and you had to hang up the phone if you were waiting on another important call.

Now, life comes at us at lightning speed: social media, text messages, streaming TV. While convenient, it can also make us think the answers to our problems are supposed to be instant—and this can prevent us from learning how to cope.

This can also be isolating. So much of life is lived online; many kids hardly spend time outside. They play video games all day, and their connection with others is mostly virtual. Or they spend hours watching their peers live large on Instagram and they feel like they're failures who don't measure up.

Another aspect of their social feeds may show them violence and despair that can be overwhelming. That's another reason I believe so many of our young people are struggling, and some are even taking their own lives. They see so much more than they're ready for. They're burning out and crying out.

Angela and I have worked hard to make sure our children maintain full lives offline. They play sports. In the summer, they're enrolled in camps far away from home where they learn to be resilient and to support, as well as depend on, their peers.

My children are wrapped in love. Bronwyn and Slater are blessed to live in a nice home, in a safe neighborhood, with parents who are fortunate enough to earn a good income. But all that doesn't mean that they are immune from stress or struggle. I know that it's easy for things to spin out of control. If they don't do well on a test, if they don't make the team, if they have a crush on someone and the affection isn't returned. Any of those things—all of those things—can leave them uncertain, anxious, or depressed.

We as parents, as teachers, as grown-ups in the neighborhood, have to talk to young people and let them know if there's a problem that won't let them sleep, a depressive thought that's grabbed hold and won't let go, they can always come talk to us.

In 2019, Slater and Bronwyn were both accepted to Southern California's equivalent of Country Day. I remembered my own experience, leaving behind my neighborhood and the local schools for private schools far away. I remembered how my parents didn't check to see how I was doing. And I knew that, with my children, I had to handle things differently.

They naturally were worried about leaving their friends, and I told them, it was true that their new school would become the center of their world and they might never see some of their old friends again. That's the way it was when you took a giant step into your future. You had to lose some things. It was scary. It might hurt.

Sure enough, the transition was very difficult. They're both smart kids, but they began to doubt themselves. Brownyn, in particular, began to struggle academically. Then, she and Slater had to deal with the disruption sparked by the pandemic, which prevented them from getting to know their new schoolmates in person.

The backdrop of their adjustment was the terrible news popping up constantly on their cell phones. They watched a violent mob break into the nation's Capitol, and they saw folks who looked like them being attacked by brutal police officers and so-called vigilantes.

"This is a terrible time," they'd say.

"Babies," I'd respond, "it's always been this way. My generation had Vietnam and the draft. You all had to live under Trump, but we had the presidencies of Richard Nixon and Ronald Reagan. You had COVID-19 but we had the beginning of AIDS. These are your trials. And your children will have theirs."

Needless to say, that wasn't particularly reassuring.

Angela and I were having difficulty calming them. We wanted to get our children help. So I told them about my own counseling journey—how their grandma encouraged me to seek it out after their grandfather killed himself. I told them how everybody needs a mental tune-up now and then and that was nothing to be embarrassed about.

We got Brownyn help first. We told her that the therapist would be her choice because we wanted her to spend time with someone she really liked talking to. Our church had a counseling center, but Bronwyn wanted to go to a place where no one knew her. Finally, we were referred to a psychologist, and she and Bronwyn clicked.

The gift of therapy—one of many—is that it brings all the problems and solutions to light. The therapist quickly determined that there was something else going on with our daughter, that she might have some learning disabilities and should be assessed. That was another health check we weren't familiar with.

It turned out that our daughter had ADHD. At her previous school, where the regimen was not as rigorous, she'd been able to manage it and excel so no one knew. But with her new school's tougher curriculum, the ADHD began to cause her problems. Once we identified it and she learned new ways to work with it, she felt empowered and began to do well again academically. I am now a fervent believer that all our young people need not only mental health checks but learning assessments because we all process things differently, and when that's not understood, it can lead to their being underestimated by others, and losing confidence in themselves.

Then it was our son's turn to get counseling. He was more reluctant.

"I don't want to, Daddy!" he said, when I told him his mother and I felt he needed to talk to someone.

I told him that we'd do it together. I'd go in there with him, though eventually he would need to go it alone because this was his time, his space, to share and speak about whatever he wanted. I also explained to him that this was just the beginning, that life would be full of difficult, stressful moments. If he thought things were complicated now, just add a relationship to the equation, or a child or two.

I also talked again about what therapy had meant to me. I told him how it changed my life, and how it's very important you go with the person you connect with, that you find your Dr. K. He ultimately decided to see a Black male psychologist recommended by Bronwyn's counselor.

When I was growing up, young Black men weren't going to therapy. And if they went off to school, or the military, they couldn't come back home when they needed a mental health break. You had to stay gone. Shoot, your bedroom might not even be there anymore.

"Where you gonna sleep?" your parents might ask. "Your room's an office now."

When my girlfriend broke up with me and I was heartbroken over Christmas, my parents were concerned but there was no way they were going to let me take time off from Harvard. I would have to pull it together and barrel through.

But we have more information than our parents had. We have

no excuse to deal with situations the way that they, their parents, or their grandparents did. If we know better, we must do better, and so it's important to encourage our young people to give voice to their pain and to get guidance to sift through it.

Thankfully, both our young people got to where they needed to be emotionally pretty quickly, particularly our son. He started out going to therapy every other week, then once a month, and finally only when he felt he needed it.

But Angela and I have let him and Bronwyn know that therapy can be one of their touchstones, always. And no matter how grown they get, how far they travel, they can always come back home.

The Mental Health Crisis

"He has issues."

"He's out of pocket."

"He's wildin'."

Those are just a few of the phrases young people toss around on social media to describe a peer who's acting out or withdrawing due to some type of emotional distress. The irony is the very platforms that they're using to label folks are the very spaces that are making so many young men anxious, afraid, depressed, and suicidal.

Social media. Reality TV. They're supposedly instant snapshots of real life. But there's nothing real about them. They are full of people living out a façade, pushing out portraits they believe present their best selves. And they leave the other young people peering in feeling inadequate.

Social media platforms also give the broader world unmitigated access to young people that was unheard of in previous generations. That's why cyberbullying is so different and uniquely devastating. Before, you had to find a way to reach your target. Now, people can harass someone else around the clock through their devices. That makes the assault so much more intense, so much more immediate—it can feel like there's no escape.

Screens also provide cover to trolls and others in attack mode, enabling them to heighten their cruelty. That's not to say people haven't always been brutal to one another. Of course they have, to an often horrifying and deadly end. But we live in a moment where an entire political party has made coarseness and bigotry its brand. Good behavior and etiquette have been eroded, and the type of actions that for a time were done in the shadows are now done unapologetically in the light.

That means if you are a young Black man, who voices an opinion, makes a joke, or simply innocently shows your face in a profile picture, screen shot, or video, the abuse you receive can be fierce. The racial slurs can be fast and furious, the stereotypes can form a thread that stretches a mile long. The trolling may demand that you take back whatever you said that indicated you feel 100 percent as human as the person attacking you. There are no sheets. They're not showing their ugliness in a secret chat. Their bigotry is flaunted out in the open for anybody and everybody to see.

And then there's the nauseating, never-ending loop of clips showing Black men being beaten and murdered by police. The video of Ahmaud Arbery out for a jog literally being hunted and running for his life as if he were a character in a video game, by bigots who displayed an unapologetic entitlement to say who they think belongs where, demonstrated what could happen to a Black man who didn't stay in his place.

That is again why language is so important. It is important that Black men find the words to acknowledge and describe their pain. It is important that you are able to verbalize your rage in a way that is not destructive to yourselves or others. And it is important to frame your trauma in a way that is truthful and liberating.

That's why I suggested Courtney stop saying that his father and godson committed suicide.

I talked with him about changing his language because you "commit" a crime, and suicide is not that. It's an act of desperation. It may be an act that comes out of anger and deep despair. But it's no more a crime than death from a heart attack or a stroke.

"Commit" implies an intentionality. For people who die by suicide, it was anything but intentional. I don't mean that the person didn't take action. They did, but there was no healthy intention behind it. They were trying to escape despair, grief, or a life they've decided is beyond repair. The only crime may be the terrible acts they may feel were committed against them. Crimes of the soul. The Soul Murder and the crimes of racism or emotional, physical, or sexual violence. Suicide happens when that person has reached the end of their rope and cannot envision some other way out.

Saying someone committed suicide also implies that the person was fully functioning mentally prior to ending their life. When someone takes their own life, especially if they have experienced extreme anguish or suffering at the hands of another, the ability to process cognitively and chemically is significantly diminished. That's especially true for those who are young, like Courtney's godson.

He was only twenty-three. Research has shown that the brain is still developing until a person is at least twenty-five years old—meaning impulse control hasn't fully been established. The same reflex that may lead a young man, feeling disrespected or hurt, to take a gun and shoot someone else may cause him to turn that gun on himself. Outsiders looking at either act may wonder, *What was he thinking?* But the answer, most likely, is that he *wasn't* thinking. Thinking means intentionally slowing down, quieting the torment, rage, embarrassment, humiliation, and despair. When your mind isn't healthy or fully developed, there may be moments when that's nearly impossible to do.

Usually those who take their own lives don't really want to die. We must reframe the common, incorrect belief that the person was a coward. What they needed, what they wanted, was relief. You don't blame someone for being in despair, for thinking they're never going to be cut a break and the only balm they can find is to leave the planet. Contrary to the false assumption that a person who kills himself sought the easy way out, it is really more likely that the person spent months or even years living in torment, and often in silence. They are not saying to life that they are done. They feel that life was done with them a long time ago.

WHAT'S GOING ON?

Suicide is the second leading cause of death of children between 10 and 14 and adults between 25 and 34, and the number three cause for those between 15 and 24, according to the National Institute of Mental Health, which cited 2020 reports from the Centers for Disease Control and Prevention.

Specifically, it was also the number three cause of death among Black people between the ages of 15 and 25 in 2019, according to the *Annual Review of Public Health*'s report "The Recent Rise of Suicide Mortality in the United States."[*]

---

[*] Gonzalo Martínez-Alés et al., "The Recent Rise of Suicide Mortality in the United States." *Annual Review of Public Health*, Vol. 43:99–116, April 2022. https://www.annualreviews.org/doi/10.1146/annurev-publhealth-051920-123206.

Young Black people already deal with adverse childhood experiences at a far greater rate than other youths, with 61% of Black American children being exposed to such potentially traumatic events as compared to 40% of white youths, according to the Center for Child Counseling.* A 2021 report from the U.S. Surgeon General also noted that children being raised in poverty were two to three times more likely to develop mental health challenges than young people who were more affluent.† Black Americans comprised 23.8% of the poor in the United States in 2019 though they made up 13.2% of the population, according to the U.S. Census Bureau.‡ Then in 2020, the world was engulfed by a once-in-a-century health crisis. Between the COVID-19 pandemic and the pressures and bullying that can come through social media, young people in particular in the last few years have been immersed in a near perfect storm of factors that make their states of mind particularly fragile. The mental health crisis among young people is severe enough that Vivek H. Murthy, the U.S. Surgeon General, issued an advisory in 2021 that noted the constellation of pressures youths and young adults are facing as well as suggestions

---

* Kerry Jamieson, "ACEs and Minorities." Center for Child Counseling, Palm Beach Gardens, FL, Dec. 13, 2018. https://www.centerforchildcounseling.org /aces-and-minorities/#:~:text=Children%20of%20different%20races%20 and,to%2040%25%20of%20white%20children.

† The U.S. Surgeon General's Advisory, "Youth Mental Health Prior to the COVID-19 Pandemic," *Protecting Youth Mental Health*. Office of the Surgeon General. U.S. Department of Health and Human Services, 2021. https://www.ncbi.nlm.nih.gov/books/NBK575985/.

‡ John Creamer, "Inequalities Persist Despite Decline in Poverty For All Major Race and Hispanic Origin Groups." U.S. Census Bureau, Sept. 15, 2020. https://www.census.gov/library/stories/2020/09/poverty-rates-for-blacks -and-hispanics-reached-historic-lows-in-2019.html.

for how parents, communities, and various systems can offer support.[*]

Beyond the crises and social phenomena distressing so many, whatever their ethnicity or gender, Black boys and men face many other challenges. These challenges can range from the seemingly small to the significant, from being hit with one too many of life's daily disappointments, to being physically violated and breaking under the trauma.

Friends and fans were shocked in 2022 when Stephen "tWitch" Boss died by suicide in a Southern California motel. The forty-year-old dancer, actor, and DJ on *The Ellen DeGeneres Show* was also a husband and the father of three children.

"It's heartbreaking to hear that someone who brought so much joy to a room, was hurting so much behind closed doors," Justin Timberlake wrote in a tweet shortly after Boss's death. "You just never know what someone is really going through."[†]

What brings someone to the brink of despair is profoundly personal. One man may be hurt when a romantic relationship ends but feel he can continue on, while another may not be able to fathom life without his vanished partner. A lost job, a bad health diagnosis, or public embarrassment may all feel, depending on the individual, like a bridge too far to cross.

And then there are facets of who you are that you might find difficult to accept. When you look in the mirror and

---

[*] The U.S. Surgeon General's Advisory, *Protecting Youth Mental Health.* https://www.hhs.gov/sites/default/files/surgeon-general-youth-mental-health-advisory.pdf.

[†] Justin Timberlake, @jtimberlake. Twitter, Dec. 14, 2022. https://twitter.com/jtimberlake/status/1603124478044577793?lang=en.

start to really glimpse your full self, your sexual identity may become clear. Perhaps you realize you are gay or non-binary. If you are surrounded by people who are not tolerant, this invalidation can make you feel judged and hopeless. Homosexuality is still too often stigmatized in the Black community, and when a young man's sexual orientation is rejected, pathologized, or demonized, it may lead him not only to self-medicate with alcohol, drugs, or sex, but also to soothe his feelings of rejection with thoughts of death.

Suicide and suicidal ideation can also be rooted in profound rage. Death can feel like the ultimate payback, a way to punish those who were unwilling to see you for all you were, or who filled you with fear, ignored your talent, or disrespected your being.

Being able to voice not only the truth of who you are, but what makes you feel angry or fearful, is essential because it enables you to feel and express all that makes you human. If we encourage Black men to talk, to say something horrible happened to them—if they encourage each other to express these things, that someone broke their heart or that they are tired of being told they aren't good enough because they are inside a Black skin—they will be able to exhale. It is critical that Black boys and men be able to say out loud, that yes, they are angry, yes, they are sad, and yes, they may be afraid.

I AM MY BROTHER'S KEEPER

About eight years ago, Kenney, a young man who was like my nephew, was killed just two weeks shy of his twenty-fifth birthday.

He was in a motorcycle accident, and of course the pain of the tragedy was immeasurable. I was asked by his mother, my dear friend, to deliver the eulogy.

Amid the packed pews were Kenney's friends. They happened to be on the richer end of the Black palette—mocha, mahogany, and shades in between. They were gorgeous and absolutely extraordinary.

They took turns paying tribute to their friend, Kenney, and they also spoke honestly about being young, dark-complexioned Black men living in America.

They spoke of a trip they'd all taken across the country one summer on Amtrak. They were worried about their safety and so as the others slept, one member of the group would stay awake, keeping watch. Someone literally "stayed woke," not according to the weaponized and demonized definition imposed by the far right, but in the way Black people who originated the phrase intended. You had to watch out for bigots and the violence that could come from them or the institutions they created. You had to stay alert so you could protect yourself and all those you cared about.

The testimonies of Kenney's friends remind me of another story I heard in the wake of the murders of George Floyd and Ahmaud Arbery. There was a young Black man in Nashville, whose neighborhood had shifted from being largely Black to white. Neighborhood watch platforms began to give reports about sightings of suspicious Black men, and this young brother became afraid to go for a walk or to even leave his house. He voiced his fears on social media, and his community, Black and white, neighbor and stranger, rallied to his side. They told him, "Come out of the house. We will walk with you." And so, one day, they did.

On the one hand, it is heartbreaking that these young men had to live with such terror. That they had to keep watch while others slept or utter the truth that they were too afraid to leave their front porch during this moment of racial backlash. But in each of those stories, I see strength, courage, and solidarity.

The young man who was afraid to go for a walk expressed his fear and accepted support. The amazing young men at Kenney's service spoke to what it is like to be afraid, but also to what it's like to have each other's backs. They spoke to the comfort that comes from knowing that someone will stay awake so you can rest. That someone will keep watch so you can replenish the strength you'll need to stay awake when it's your brother's turn to sleep.

They didn't cancel their trip. But they also weren't naïve. They didn't posture or hide behind a façade of hypermasculinity. They knew that to be young Black men traveling across this country, entering unknown, white spaces to eat, to sightsee, to swim, there could be danger. They watched out for each other. And they refused to be silent about what they did, and why they needed to do it.

There's a beautiful lesson in that for every Black man and boy. Look for those who will walk with you, who will surround you and make an effort to keep you safe. Look for that person who will keep watch while you rest. We all need someone who will stay awake so we can be restored. Then, when we are awakened, we can stand vigil for them.

Tell Somebody

It is also important to be vigilant when it comes to recognizing signs of your own emotional distress, particularly if it's leading you to consider ending your life. Maybe you are telling yourself, "I want to die," and thinking about how you can make that happen. Maybe you have created a script justifying how much better off everyone else will be—your coworkers, your kids, your friends—if you are no longer here, disappointing them or making them worry.

If you are having these kinds of thoughts, don't isolate yourself. Tell someone how you are feeling. And if you don't have anyone you feel you can confide in, call 988 (in the U.S.) to contact the Suicide & Crisis Lifeline. People taking those calls are trained, and often in recovery from their own depression and suicidal thoughts. The crisis line can be a safe space where you feel heard, supported, and not judged.

SIGNS AND SOLUTIONS FOR THE PEOPLE WHO LOVE YOU

What signs should those who love Black men and boys look for if they fear their loved one is running out of hope and considering ending it all?

Often, a person contemplating suicide will tell multiple people that they are struggling emotionally. We just may not want to hear it, since it hurts us when someone we love is suffering. We don't want to believe it. We're unsure how to help. So we may decide instead to shut them down. We may say, *Why would you think about that when you have so much to offer?* We may say, *I could never live without you,* or perhaps we act like we didn't hear a word.

We may not mean to, but when we dismiss or ignore our loved ones' cries for help, we render them invisible. We risk increasing their feelings of isolation and sadness because we can't tolerate their suffering and our terror and feelings of helplessness.

If our friend or son or brother or husband has gotten to a point where he wants to take his own life and his efforts to talk about the reasons why are ignored, he may eventually go silent and finally follow through with his plan. He had the words, yet like someone who speaks a foreign language but is discouraged from using it, he will eventually lose the ability to articulate what he is feeling.

And because a suicidal person's cognition is already compromised, owing either to their emotional struggles or because they are young and coping with an underdeveloped brain, they can convince themselves that people would be better off if they are gone. Yes, they understand, people will be sad. Yes, their parents will be upset. But their loved ones, they reason, may also be relieved. After all, their loved ones didn't want to hear what they had to say about their distress anyway. They imagine that those who love them will be liberated from this unimaginable emotional storm. With their death, everyone can get a break.

Others may encourage our troubled loved one to simply pray. We might truly believe that's the answer, but we may also suggest prayer because it gets us off the hook. It's easier to tell them to tell their troubles to God than to take the time ourselves to sit and listen, and to feel our own helplessness.

As hard as it might be, we must be the mirror that reflects back to them that they are not crazy. Instead of giving them platitudes, a scolding, or simply instructing them to pray, ask them to tell you more. How often are they thinking about suicide? What is their plan?

It can feel uncomfortable. But being able to sit and listen to someone tell you how badly they hurt can be key to helping them get help and saving their life.

Conversely, if we don't listen to our loved one who is considering suicide, they may stop telling us how badly they feel. We really need to pay attention to someone who was figuratively bleeding out in front of us and, all of a sudden, the bleeding stops. We may want to move on, relieved that they seem to be doing better because they're not talking about their pain or their longing to not be here anymore. But just like a hemorrhage doesn't stop on its own, it's rare that the distress that made someone feel suicidal will just go away without deliberate treatment and intervention.

I know people want to believe. They talk about a brother who went to church, or a nephew who prayed for hours and had an epiphany that erased his emotional pain. But while their loved one may have felt lifted in the moment, that's likely just a Band-Aid on a gaping wound. Prayer can be soothing, but for someone who is contemplating suicide, additional support and treatment are usually needed.

If someone is talking about their suicidal thoughts, and then they just stop, pay attention. If they are suddenly sleeping through the night, taking phone calls from friends, and no longer picking at their plate—essentially doing things they had been avoiding—you may want to ask even more questions.

They might have stopped talking because they're going to enact their plan soon and so they are relaxed. They might be returning to their old routine because they know they won't have to endure their pain much longer. We need to remain vigilant.

Seek Support

It's not just your suicidal loved one who needs support. You will likely need a shoulder to lean on as well to deal with the pain that is ignited when your son, nephew, or partner is in such agony. But the stigma around suicide often makes that hard to do. There is so much misguided shame that when a loved one contemplates or attempts suicide, that becomes the next family secret. We don't lean on our neighbors. We don't reach out to our relatives or a religious leader to tell him or her that this is happening and we don't know what to do.

You need your own compassionate solid reinforcement in order to help your loved one get the mental health help they deserve and require. That's not the person who says suicide is a sin. That's not the cousin who questions why your boyfriend, who's handsome and affluent, or your son who is smart and has so much to look forward to, would think for a moment about taking his life. You don't need someone who will shut you down.

You want to partner with a professional or a friend or a community that is able to deal compassionately with a situation that makes all of us feel frightened and helpless. And you want to seek the support of someone who

> understands that mental health struggles are something
> that to some degree every one of us will experience. You
> can call the Suicide & Crisis Lifeline for your loved one,
> and for yourself. Contact a community mental health cen-
> ter, or if you have a primary care physician, ask them to
> refer you to resources that they can recommend.

LIFE ISN'T VIRTUAL

Your elders must also be willing to talk to young people about their own emotional struggles, modeling the ways to wellness.

Courtney, for instance, passed it on. Though his parents' generation often lacked the language to speak about mental health, or perhaps lacked the permission to proactively tend to it, his mother actively encouraged him to get counseling and sought it out for herself after Courtney's father's suicide. Courtney, in turn, shared the power of therapy with his children, telling them about his own experience, and how going to therapy was an act of strength and courage.

Your parents or caregivers probably taught you how to cross the street and how to clean up after yourself. Someone reminded you to button up your coat so you wouldn't catch a cold, and someone probably wanted you home before dark.

Your emotional well-being is no less important, but par-ents don't always attend to this. They are individuals too. They don't have it all together and can't model perfection in that area because it's not possible. This is something essential for young people to understand. As Courtney did with his kids, and within the pages of this book, revealing our tough road helps others realize that as long as we walk through the world, we will be works in progress, learning and growing as we go. And constantly doing a self-examination, expressing how we feel, and asking for support are really what matters.

When you fill the void with your personal stories, you no longer need to rely so much on the often false images and negativity that flood social media, those that show your peers living impossibly perfect lives or cyberbullies picking on others. You can be reminded of the particular affirmation that comes from live human connection. Of the beauty of hearing another's voice, of sitting face-to-face, or of being in the same room with someone you care about and who cares about you. And you'll likely want to put down the phone, set aside the iPad, and take a break.

It's not easy to ignore social media when so much of the world lives online. But there are young public figures who are being vocal about their mental health struggles and the need to turn down the volume. Tom Holland, the most recent star of the *Spider-Man* film franchise, announced in the summer of 2022 that he was taking a hiatus from Twitter and Instagram because they were "overstimulating" and "overwhelming." "It's very detrimental to my mental state," he said in an Instagram video, "so I decided, to take a step back and delete the app."

You don't have to abandon social media entirely. When tapped into selectively, it can serve a great purpose, providing information about how to find mental health and other forms of support. As of 2023, TikTok in particular has actually become a place of healing for many young people dealing with death and loss who post videos to bond with others using hashtags like #griefjourney and #grieftok.

But to seize the depth and the breadth of life, its difficulties as well as its joys, we can't just observe it through screens. We need to dive into it, taste it, experience it, physically as well as emotionally.

So many of our young Black men don't realize that they have the right to hurt, and also the right to heal. The more separated you are from the idea that you are entitled to be whole, the more silent you might be about your suffering. So you may be labeled as crazy instead of simply human, or described as violent without others acknowledging your justifiable anger, and this prevents you from obtaining clarity. Being able to sound off on what you're feeling is essential.

Black man, you are right to be afraid when you are pulled over by a police officer. You are right to worry when you enter a store, check into a hotel, or drive down a narrow road in an unfamiliar, colorless place. Yes, something might go terribly wrong though you've done absolutely nothing to deserve it. If you are living in the same world that I'm in, then, my brother, I hope you have some good fear that will make you pragmatic and keep you alive.

We also know that, on top of that, there are just the daily struggles that we all must handle. Making sure our children are physically healthy and well cared for. Navigating work. Maintaining a positive relationship with our spouse or partner. Keeping on top of schoolwork. It's a lot. It can make you scream. And so, sometimes, you should.

But know that there are others who will walk with you. Who will keep watch. Who will listen. Pain may endureth for a night. It may come and go and come back again. But there will always be a morning, you deserve to claim it for yourself.

WHAT TO TAKE AWAY

* **Ask for help.** Tell a loved one if you're feeling suicidal and don't let them brush you off. Keep telling someone until they listen, your pain deserves to be heard.
* **Other resources.** Call the Suicide & Crisis Lifeline at 988 if needed, which can connect you to a crisis counselor at any time of the day. Seek out a therapist. Medication may also be necessary and helpful, and can be prescribed by a physician or mental health professional. The National Alliance on Mental Illness suggests reaching out to the National Treatment Referral Helpline 800-662-HELP (4357) or findtreatment.samhsa.gov for guidance to affordable mental health services. Additionally, Mental Health America offers online screenings for a range of conditions, including depression, anxiety, and self-injury. You can go to www.mhascreening.org to do a self-assessment that can help you figure out if you need to seek mental health support.
* **Say it out loud.** There's no shame in being afraid, or angry or worried. Give voice to it in safe places, and with safe and trustworthy people. You'll no doubt find that many others in your life feel the same.
* **Take a social media break.** Social media can be a lifeline at times, connecting you to others with similar experiences or offering support. But if you're becoming overwhelmed, tell your followers and friends

you're at least temporarily signing off. Take the time to interact and connect with those you choose who, even if they disagree with you, know how to do so respectfully.

✳ **Parents, be role models.** When it comes to tending to mental health, let the young people in your world know if you've pursued therapy. Acknowledge that you also struggle, and that everyone has emotional work to do. Preaching doesn't help. Being compassionately present does.

CHAPTER 6

How to Lose
(On Death and Dying)

"Ain't nothing wrong with talking about death. That's part of life. You gonna die. I'm gonna die. Everybody gonna die."

—TROY MAXSON, *FENCES*

When my father killed himself, my mother's decision to stay put gave me a lesson in how to keep going.

My sister and I began talking about where Mom could move because we thought there was no way she could stay in the house on Appoline. There would be too many bad memories. How could she ever go into that TV room again and not see my father's body lying there on the floor? Dad had filled that house with his vibrancy when he was alive, and his absence in death left nothing but questions and shadows.

No. Mommy couldn't stay there, we decided. Maybe we could find her a condo in a nice neighborhood just outside Detroit.

But when we talked to our mother about leaving, she said she wouldn't go.

"I'm staying in this house," she said defiantly. "I'm going to work out with my Lord whatever needs to be worked out."

My mother taught me so much in my life. She brought home books from her job at the library when I was just a toddler to teach me how to read. She helped me recognize the call of a cardinal and how it differed from the chirp of a blackbird. And she taught me that you could lean on the Lord, and a therapist too.

But her choice to stay in our family home taught Cecilie and me something else. Just as she was being a role model, encouraging us to follow in her footsteps and get counseling, she was also teaching us that life is about rebounding. Life is about pivoting. Just like in a football game, or on the basketball court, when you fall, you have to get up. And if you can't stand on your own, lean on whoever you need to until you can.

Therapy gave our family a place to take our grief, so it didn't just consume all of the space in the house on Appoline, at my sister's home in Germany, or inside my tiny apartment back in New York. We could talk about our sadness, so it didn't feel quite so heavy. We had a space to ponder why Dad did what he did, why we didn't see it coming, and even if we had, whether there was anything we could have done.

I think each of us had our own set of questions. Maybe, I thought, if I wasn't away from home so much, from the time I was young, Dad would have hesitated, given me a call, and changed his mind. I'm sure my mother, aware of her husband's painful childhood, wondered if she could have pushed and probed a little more.

And then there was Cecilie, who'd had her own very public mental health battle ever since high school. She was the one among us who'd actually been going to counseling for years. She took medication daily to steady her mood. And, I learned after my father's death, she, too, had contemplated suicide.

My parents, knowing her dark thoughts, worked with Cecilie's therapist to give her reasons to stay.

"Stay here for your mother," they told her. "Stay here for your brother. But please. Just stay."

So, for Cecilie, it was even more jarring to realize Dad had done what he'd fought so hard to keep her from doing. Now, if those terrible thoughts ever returned, she had an even bigger incentive to ward them off.

She had to be here, not only to see how her life played out, but for Mom and for me. After all, we had endured the pain of Dad's suicide. How could we possibly survive another?

———

As I prepared for life after Harvard, I auditioned for the Yale School of Drama. And I got in.

Lloyd Richards was the Drama School's dean. An elegant man with copper skin and wire-rimmed glasses, Lloyd was born in Canada, but grew up in Detroit. He was a lion in the theater world long before he came to Yale, becoming the first Black person to direct a play on Broadway when he helmed Lorraine Hansberry's *A Raisin in the Sun*. He also worked with the great South African playwright Athol Fugard. But Lloyd's most enduring partnership was with the great August Wilson, who staged six of his plays at Yale, including *The Piano Lesson*, *Ma Rainey's Black Bottom*, and *Fences*.

I was getting cast in a lot of productions on campus, because of my look and my acting chops—I looked like Joe College, the quintessential young American man so long as you didn't think that the All-American boy had to be blue-eyed and blond. And I was super focused in class. But when I saw the casting flyer for *Fences*, and the description of Cory Maxson, a teenage football star, I didn't see myself in him. Even though I'd been an athlete, I figured they'd want a burly guy the audience could instantly relate to. So I looked forward to seeing the play knowing that I wouldn't be in it.

Then, several days later, my girlfriend and classmate at the time told me to go look at the casting board, and there I saw my name listed for the role of Cory. Once again, my classroom work had won me a great role. I was in shock.

Suddenly, I was performing alongside these titans of acting. James Earl Jones played Troy Maxson, Cory's father. There was also Frankie Faison, still a great friend to this day, who had the role of Gabriel, Troy's mentally ill brother. Charles Brown played Cory's half brother, Lyons, and Ray Aranha was Jim Bono, Troy's good friend.

And in the midst of all those men was Mary Alice.

Mary Alice played Rose, Troy's wife and Cory's mother. But in her long career, she embodied many iconic characters, from Dr. Bessie Delany in the Broadway hit *Having Our Say*, to "The Oracle" in *The Matrix* film series.

I was intimidated. It was impossible not to be. Here were all these legends and I was a graduate student who half the time didn't know what I was doing. Sure, I could deliver an emotional punch with a line. Yes, I had "the look." But I was green.

I wanted to keep learning, and I'm a master of observation. Watching James and Frankie and Charles and Mary Alice, I learned how to work. I became an actor.

Eventually we took the play on the road, Lloyd tweaking and

polishing as we went from city to city. I checked in with my acting elders constantly, asking in between matinees and evening performances, over lunch and during cast dinners if I was doing okay.

"It's all right, Courtney," they'd say if I missed a mark or fumbled a line. "It's all right."

Always, they took care of me. Always, they showed me love. They gave me kindness. They were family.

After playing across the United States, *Fences* became one of the many August Wilson plays to make it to Broadway. It went on to win the Pulitzer Prize and to sweep the Tony Awards in 1987. Night after night, we went onstage, me continuing to study, James, Mary Alice, and Frankie continuing to teach.

And the lessons weren't just about acting.

Though I was nominated for a Tony Award for my performance as Cory, when it came time to re-up our contracts, most of us weren't offered raises. Only the show's major stars, James and Mary Alice, would see their salaries go up. And there was no negotiating. It was take it or leave it. I was ready to go.

Frankie, Charles, and Ray took me aside. "Courtney," they said. "Stay."

"But..." I blustered.

"Courtney," they repeated, "it's Mary Alice's and James's time. It's not yours. That's why they got paid."

Sometimes, as you let the mud clear, a little bit splatters in your face. I had to sit in my feelings for a few days, but I ultimately decided to stick with the show. I'm so glad I did because eventually I got to the other side of that youthful hurt. I waited long enough for my bruised ego to heal. And now, decades later, when I'm often the one receiving top billing, I'm able to pass that wisdom on to the next impatient young actor.

"You'll be all right," I tell them. "Stick it out. Keep going. And you'll be glad you did when you come out on the other side."

———————

Mary Alice and I grew especially close during our days doing *Fences*. She and I used to say that the hardest thing about that moment in time was getting to the theater. If we could just get to the Forty-Sixth Street (now the Richard Rodgers) Theater and open the stage door, we'd be all right because our make-believe world was constant. We knew what to do. But outside that building, the world was a mess.

I continued to have inklings of doubt about whether I'd truly made the right choice staking my professional future in the fickle world of acting. And my longtime girlfriend and I were struggling. Life, meanwhile, was even harder for Mary Alice. She lost both her mother and her father during our Broadway run. I watched her, wondering how she could ever find peace, or even concentrate on her performance in the midst of such pain.

But Mary Alice showed me how. She didn't run from her emotions. She cried when she needed to and turned back to work when her tears were spent. She also accepted despite her sorrow that dying was an inescapable part of life.

My parents, who came to every opening night from California to New York, appreciated Mary Alice's presence, knowing that I was in good hands with her watching over me. And in time, Mary Alice would also nurture my wife, Angela. Long after our initial Broadway run, Angela was cast as Rose in a staging of *Fences* at the Pasadena Playhouse with Laurence Fishburne. I told her she had to call Mary Alice, and the two of them became thick as thieves.

No holiday was complete until we heard from our Mother Mary. She was an integral part of our lives, always asking after Cecilie, becoming another grandmother to Slater and Bronwyn. She sang "Happy Birthday" to each of us on our special day, and if we weren't home, she left her rich rendition in a voice mail. I actually preferred that to being there to get the call because it meant I could listen to her serenade us over and over again.

Like my mother, Leslie, Mary Alice constantly taught me about the ebb and flow of life. When she retired because she no longer had the stamina to take the stage every night or to sit for hours in a trailer waiting to do a scene, it messed with her emotions. She was open about her battle with depression, about getting on medication and struggling to get the dosage right. I took my turn as nurturer, escorting Mary Alice from her apartment in Manhattan to the Christian Cultural Center in Brooklyn for some literal soul food dished out by the powerful Pastor A. R. Bernard. I tried to give Mary Alice as much support as she'd always given me.

"It's all right, Mary Alice," I'd tell her. "It's all right."

And Angela and I were overjoyed to see Mary Alice come through the darkness. By 2022, she was ready to party again. She was going to the theater, enjoying being in the audience, and content with her decision to no longer be onstage. She knew this was her new season, and she embraced and relished her role as a fan as well as a master teacher. Mary Alice was also excited about seeing James Earl Jones receive the rare honor of having a Broadway theater named after him, like our beloved August Wilson years before.

Then on July 28, I got the call. Mary Alice had passed away. I called James. "She was so kind and warm, wasn't she,

Courtney," he said in that unmistakable voice, now husky with grief.

"Yes," I said. "She was."

———————

Mary Alice died of natural causes. That's a way of dying that people have no trouble putting in the obituary. Suicide, however, is something many people want to hide.

But not me. I didn't lie and say my dad died of a heart attack or a disease. Suicide to me wasn't shameful. Maybe because I had no real sense of it. It was like bungee jumping or drag racing, something I would never think to do. That's not to say I'm stronger or better than the many people who do think about suicide. It just wasn't part of my consciousness.

So I didn't deny that my father killed himself. But I remained shocked that he'd done it. And the most devastating fact of all was however he went out, I had to learn to go on and live without him.

That's why catching my dreams became so important. It gave me something to focus on. I knew when I went to sleep that I was going to be working.

Trying to capture the rhythm of my dream life meant that I was taking care of myself. I was trying to heal. I became aware of how I often lived life on offense and made decisions impulsively. My scribbled-down dreams filled at least one journal a month, cover to cover, for four years. I highlighted which ones I wanted to discuss with Dr. K in red ink and even created tables of contents—"Bottom," "Natalie Cole," "Country Day."

When I began to bob and weave from grief, or sink into despair, I'd remember what came to me in my sleep. I'd search for the guidance my dreams gave to my life, and I'd regain my bearings. Then, when I was steady, I could be still and feel again. Over time, I could think about my dad without my knees buckling. I could remember him, and instead of breaking down, I'd smile. I'd always regret he didn't get the help he needed and deserved. My dad was worthy of care and relief in life, but he died before understanding that death was not his only option to find this peace. Still, I began to accept the fact I couldn't rewind time.

My job was on Broadway, but my real work was done after dark when I was learning myself. That became the center of my life. And during those years, therapy helped me even more than my faith, because while I was always drawn to God, I was still searching for my spiritual home. Dr. K stood in the gap for me. Just like the therapist who talked to my sister, and the psychologist who worked with my mother. She stood in the breach so I didn't end up like my father, lost and without hope.

But Dr. K also let me know that she was trying to wean me off her. She was helping me get to a place where I could do this work for myself, by myself. In a sense, she'd walked with me through the valley of the shadow of death and stayed with me until I could find the strength to pull myself out of there on my own.

———

Fences is so deep within me, I recite its lines even now like a prayer. And death is a thread that runs through it.

Troy talks about how he fought death and won. He tells the truth about how it will come for everyone, but he isn't scared. And in the end, death does indeed come calling and Troy has no choice but to succumb.

"Ain't nothing wrong with talking about death," he says. "That's part of life. Everybody gonna die. You gonna die, I'm gonna die. Hell, we all gonna die. "

"I looked up one day and death was marching right at me. Like soldiers on parade. The army of death marching straight at me!"

"Death ain't nothin' but a fastball on the outside corner. An' you KNOW what I'll do to that!"

Ain't nothing wrong with talking about death. And yet so many of us can't do it. It hurts too much to think about. We don't want to face how much we miss the person who's gone. Or maybe we're afraid of it knocking on our door.

But we've got to speak on it. When we do, we can celebrate our loved ones as well as mourn them. We can look at who and what we have with a renewed appreciation because we know there will be a day when it all disappears. We can let the next person, and the next person, and the one after that know that sorrow is an emotion we will all inevitably feel, but along with sadness and grieving, there can be rejoicing and gratitude too.

I can remember how Angela and I would go visit Mary Alice, or the legendary acting couple Ossie Davis and Ruby Dee and just let their wisdom wash over us, hoping it would always be like this but knowing one day we'd wake up and find that they were gone. Ruby and Ossie. Mary Alice and Lloyd. Sidney Poitier and Cicely Tyson. One by one, all those giants have left the world. And one day, Angela and I will follow. That's the river of life. That's the way that goes, just like Gabriel said when he blew his horn at the end of *Fences*.

That's why speaking about suicide, about loss, and about healing too, has become like a ministry for me. I eagerly share my story with anyone who will listen. My father killed himself. My godson too. My mothers, Leslie and Mary Alice, are gone. I miss them terribly. I needed therapy at times to survive. But I'm here. And while I cherish their memories, I also treasure every single breath I take, and every single day God gives me. My elders taught me about accepting the need to constantly transition, and not to be so mired in sorrow for who and what I've lost that I miss out on all the wonder and joy still lying in front of me.

———

I also understood that, to deal with loss, there are certain things you have to let go. Like judging the person who's gone, or yourself for not doing something different when they were here. When you judge, you become angry. What you judge, you can't explore, examine, or learn from. You cast blame or feel superior. You carry that negative energy like a bag of boulders on your back, and it weighs down your entire existence.

I think that's why my grandfather and uncles made sure to tell me not to judge my father when we all gathered at his funeral. They didn't want me to carry that resentment. Dr. K said the same thing. To carry on with the unending grief he must have felt for his mother took resilience. It took courage. But in the end, he just couldn't overcome the loss of a parent he'd never known.

However, when our loved ones leave, when death does come calling, we can all remind each other that there will be a time when the memories of how they lived is more resonant than when—or how—they died.

One day, a few years back, I was speaking to a dear family friend, Miss Anita. She told me that her brother had called that morning and mentioned that it was the fifteenth anniversary of their father's death. But Miss Anita had forgotten. At some point she'd stopped ticking off the years.

"Courtney," she asked. "Is there something wrong with me?"

"No," I told her. "You're busy living."

And so am I. It's been more than thirty-two years since my own father died. It was on December 19, 1990. But sometimes now, I forget the date.

I told Miss Anita that our focus now is not on the drama and trauma of what happened. Our focus is on carrying out our journey, and so certain moments will recede into the shadows while other experiences come to the fore.

I know it's hard to imagine there will be a time when the death of a parent, or a sibling or a child, doesn't occupy your every thought and the pain doesn't pierce your entire being. But gradually, it may no longer be the center of your world. And that's a good thing.

It's up to each of us who've come through these valleys to teach others that they can make it out as well. And yes, there will be more grief, but with every loss, you can reach back and remember that somehow you were able to keep going. Knowing that can give you the hope you'll survive again.

Don't Feed the Beast

This is what you do with grief. You don't ignore it, but you don't feed it. And there is a difference, because what you feed grows. What you acknowledge heals.

Grief is unavoidable. Heartache and heartbreak are part of being human. And Black men, who also must watch their brothers fall victim to violence meted out by a hostile world and sometimes, tragically, by each other, endure much more than their share. Black children witnessing homicides on a regular basis are being traumatized in a way that their white counterparts are not, and thus need interventions and safe respite from the violent death angel bombarding and stealing their innocence. Death and loss may come to feel like an endless loop they can't escape, and so they may submerge their sorrow with sex, overwork, or drugs. Maybe they are so mired in denial, they numb themselves to all emotion, including happiness. And sometimes they flee their pain permanently, by taking their own lives.

But if grief is resisted, if it's minimized or ignored, it doesn't disappear. Instead, its power grows. It becomes a beast of its own. We can't outrun it. Grief is meant to be explored, understood, and even embraced from the moment we are born until we take our last breath.

So no, you can't just "get over it." Like healing, and forgiveness, grief is not finite. You may wake up one morning months after your sibling's death, finally feeling like your old self, and then the next day, your loved one's absence makes you double over in pain. That's natural. That's human. We are meant to interrogate and integrate loss into our lives like all of our other emotions and experiences.

TAKE OFF THE SUNGLASSES

In the Western World, we don't deal well with death. Many of us don't even like to say the word. We act as though being stoic in the face of it is a great achievement, something to be proud of. But how do you keep your composure when you will never see your mother again in this lifetime? How do you stay serene when you realize you will never again hear the voice of a dear friend?

Just like we explode with laughter when we hear a wonderful joke, gasp in wonder when we see a blazing sunrise, or bop with joy when our favorite song blasts through a speaker, it's important to release our sorrow too.

So cry. Cry in public. Cry out loud. Cry until you don't have a tear left to shed.

It can be hard for Black men in particular to express their grief openly. You may often feel constrained by the codes of hypermasculinity. The pressures of societal expectations, which demand that you be tough and hard, combined with the systemic oppression that has often made it more difficult for you to provide for and protect your families, make you hold on even tighter to so-called markers of manhood.

It's why at so many funerals, many of you sit in the pews wearing sunglasses. You're not only hiding your tears. As you look at that casket, you may be trying to cover up the fear that you may be next. In certain neighborhoods, after certain conflicts, you may be legitimately worried that there will be a shootout at the funeral home, at the cemetery, or at the repast.

But if you hide your tears, if you don't find the words to talk about your anxiety, if you feel that showing vulnerability makes you look weak, you are relinquishing your right to be fully human. Of course you are sad. Of course you are anxious. Of course you might be afraid. You have a birthright to all those feelings, without shame.

There's a reason why, when babies are born, they are tapped on their backside. Their cries clear their airways. Their tears express their bewilderment at their sudden arrival in this strange new world. That's what tears are, a release and a declaration.

When the Black men who are my patients and friends feel free to weep—about abandonment and sexual abuse, about illness and death—they are better able to sustain themselves and those they love. Unburdening enables them to gather the strength they need to tackle whatever task or trial is next.

Two Black fathers, Omari Maynard and Bruce McIntyre III, convene groups of Black men around the country who have lost their partners after childbirth. Bonded by tragedy, they are embracing discomfort and normalizing grief. They are bearing witness to each other's vulnerability. They are sharing and showing their tears. They are holding each other, and healing in public while raising their children as widowed black fathers.

Tears can free us, inspiring us to look within at what is causing us distress, allowing us to deal with our pain before we implode or inflict our pain on someone else. Tears are our teacher. They never lie. What are your tears teaching you?

A man who cries is demonstrating that he has access to all parts of who he is. What he likes, what he hates, who he loves, what he's lost. He is awake. He's showing up by facing his emotions. And by doing that, he will only grow.

Take off the sunglasses and cry out loud. When you do, you free yourself, and encourage others around you to release their pain as well.

OUR DEPARTED LOVED ONES ARE OUR TEACHERS

Courtney has drawn lessons not only from how his father lived, but also from how he died. He moves in his own life differently now, with more intention, with more heart, with more metabolized and integrated power.

We would never choose for any of those we love to die. But if we look at death as simply the next stage in their journey, we can accept that those whose destinies connect with ours have much to teach us and those lessons don't stop when we are no longer able to touch them. In fact, their most pertinent lessons may be found in the way they leave.

Courtney honors his father and godson by making sure that their lives and deaths by suicide will not be in vain. He has made it his mission to talk about how common suicide is, to let those whose loved ones take their own lives understand that they are not alone, and to let other Black men know there are resources they can turn to if they are contemplating suicide themselves so they can make a different choice.

I once did some work for a Fortune 100 company. A number of Black men working for the firm had died, many from suicide. I asked that each of their names be written on a poster board and placed at the front of the conference room. The reason was to make clear that, though they were dead, their suffering and their stories were not. The people at the company could take actions to make the work environment better. They could schedule conversations where people could talk about the pressures they were under in and outside the office. They could learn the signs to watch out for to determine if a person was nearing the end of their rope and seek knowledge about how to offer support.

"This," I told the people gathered together in that room, "is an opportunity."

If a loved one dies from suicide, from an overdose, from driving recklessly down an open road, don't waste time being ashamed of how they left. Don't blame yourself for what you did or didn't do. Shame is a silencer. Shame is a killer. Shame wastes precious time. Instead, think about what the messages are for us who are still living.

Perhaps for the church family of Courtney's godson, the message was that sometimes God's healing comes through medication. His parents knew that, but there might've been a grandmother in their congregation who believed therapy was the devil and the only medication anyone ever needs is prayer. But after hearing this story, maybe she started to shift her thinking. Maybe if she had a grandchild, or a neighbor in emotional distress, instead of just telling him it would be all right, or directing him to pray, she'd now encourage him to also consider talking to a therapist.

For the corporate manager whose colleague killed himself, maybe the lesson is not to berate himself for not realizing how troubled his coworker was, but to learn what to look out for next time so he can do more for another peer who is struggling emotionally.

Bring the memory of those we've lost to the front of the room, then take a seat, listen, and learn so that you can get up, go out, and live better.

ANOTHER KIND OF LOSS

If grief is hindering you, consider grief counseling. Just about everyone who loses someone may have moments when they don't want to get out of bed and face the day. But if you find yourself playing video games all day, every day, for months. If you are bingeing on exercise, sex, or drugs. If you are withdrawing socially, or conversely find yourself unable to ever be still and alone, you might want to talk to a mental health professional. You might need to sift through your grief with someone who is willing to listen. That doesn't have to be a professional therapist. It can be a good friend, a caring coach, your barber, or a neighborhood elder. But look for someone willing and able to welcome, bear witness and hold your tears.

It's also important to remember that loss comes in many forms beyond death. There is the pain of heartbreak. There is the bitter taste left when a friend betrays you. Many Black men also have to deal with the sorrow that comes from realizing they've been denied the opportunity to fulfill their dreams because of racism and other injustices.

There can be tremendous grief when you realize that you could have had a different life. It can gnaw at you, preventing you from appreciating what you have been able to attain. You may feel that you failed, that you weren't worthy of that love you yearned for and lost, or the professional goal that eluded you. Your grief can show up as depression, disconnection, resentment, or rage.

That's not to say you would necessarily have been a surgeon or a famous journalist if systemic racism hadn't been in your way. But maybe, if there were guidance counselors in your high school that taught you about the SAT, you could have gone to college. Maybe you could have owned your own business if the bank hadn't denied you a loan or only offered financing with an exorbitant interest rate, despite your good credit, simply because you were Black.

It's like when the practice of redlining was finally called out. It wasn't that most Black people didn't want to buy homes. Many of us, despite great odds, have accomplished that milestone. But some went without as banks were literally allowed to deny mortgages to those living in Black neighborhoods or even give them the funding that a white person could obtain to fix a crumbling roof or do other repairs. That Black would-be homeowner might have thought something was wrong with him, only to learn that the system, with all its levers and pulleys, was set up to make it as hard as possible for a Black person to purchase property, to hold on to it once they got it, and therefore to build and pass on generational wealth.

Of course, you grieve what might have been if racism didn't bar you from certain jobs and universities, if deliberate disinvestment in your neighborhood didn't weaken the schools you went to or deprive your community of parks and other green space. But there can also be something redemptive in recognizing that you were born capable and equipped and opportunities didn't elude you because you were unworthy, but because someone threw obstacles in your path. That awareness doesn't correct the injustice, and yes, you can and should still feel enraged or sad. But if you stop there, that anger and grief will eat you alive.

The task for you as a Black man is to take what you know now about what held you back, and make sure that knowledge doesn't become an excuse not to accomplish all that you still can achieve. Black men's indignation and pain should be acknowledged, but that doesn't have to be the end of the story. Maybe you didn't go to college right after high school because you mistakenly believed everyone getting a higher education was a genius and you were not. But you can look in the mirror and set new goals, and as you reach them, you'll inspire and motivate others who'll want to follow your lead.

You who are awakening to your own potential, you who are showing up to shape your own destiny, you who are rewriting the script in your head and crying in public without shame are ripe for claiming your joy. You can resolve that whatever injustice has obstructed your path in the past won't stand in the way of your right here, right now determination. Otherwise, those who've always wanted to deny you the chance to be your fullest self are the ones who will win.

A man named Anthony Ray Hinton was wrongly accused of two murders he didn't commit. He went to prison in 1985 and didn't walk free until almost thirty years later after a team of lawyers, including Bryan Stevenson, the great attorney and civil rights warrior, won his release in 2015. (Stevenson proclaims "that capital punishment is the stepchild of lynching.")

I've heard Mr. Hinton speak often. What he had to endure was unimaginable. But he recognizes that he can either give the systems and forces that locked him up unjustly what's left of his life, or he can figure out how to hold the memory of this terrible injustice while recognizing that the sun still shines, and he deserves perhaps more than anyone to bask in its warmth. Since his release, he has become an inspirational speaker, a writer, and in 2020, he voted for president for the first time.

So many of us get tripped up thinking we're too old to try something new, or to begin again. We get stuck on what could have been, and we spend so much time looking backward that the past becomes our present and the present becomes our future.

"I'm taking this one class when I could have been done with law school by now," you might say. But if you stay in that space, feeding that loss, then the one class you signed up for is not going to get your best effort. If you're so busy resenting that you're not further along, you might miss out on the mentorship of that professor who believes you have great potential.

As long as you're living, there is the chance for change. Time is going to pass whether you are choosing to honor yourself or not. So you might as well discover and lean into what gives you happiness and a sense of fulfillment.

Take that class, that job, that opportunity. It may not restore the previous five, ten, or twenty years that have passed, but it's a step toward your goal now. With every new moment of possibility, the pain of what you missed eases a little more. Some things in your rearview mirror might have been unfairly taken. But you don't have to allow this moment to be stolen too.

FEED YOUR SPARK, NOT YOUR SORROW

Several years ago, I was in two car accidents that messed up my body, my mental state, and my credit. If I continued

to start and end my day dwelling in the misery those accidents caused, I'd only feed my debilitation. If Courtney
languished in recriminations and regret after his father's
and godson's suicides, those tragedies would have become
the biggest part of who Courtney B. Vance is. He would be
sapped of the creativity that fuels his award-winning work
in films and on the stage. He'd miss out on the joy of raising Slater and Bronwyn and having a lifetime partnership
with Angela.

Those suicides are certainly a part of him. To a Black boy
in America, the racist move of a private school headmaster
had an impact. But Courtney has learned to let those memories sit without giving them additional energy. Yes, Black
men have been traumatized and discriminated against. You
may have been denied jobs and opportunities. But when you
dig into who you truly are, and gain insight into your interests and gifts, you feed your spark and not your sorrow.

I've seen what happens when Black men make that
choice. All of a sudden, they sit up straighter. They stride
strong into a room and have a glint in their eyes. They give
their brothers and sons the incentive to dream bigger, so
they, too, can pursue what makes them feel accomplished
and full of hope. When they get a glimpse of their true
selves mirrored by those who care for them, they remember
that they are whole not despite their emotional wounds, but
because of them.

It's a delicate balancing act, acknowledging the injuries
of yesterday or the pain of losing a loved one, while not letting it overwhelm the sweet times your life still has in store.
Ask for help. Seek out the spiritual space or group that will
mirror back how difficult your past trauma was, and also

remind you that you have a divine right to continue on and be happy. Find that therapist or friend who will not only bear witness to your struggle but also proclaim your light. With their support, you can both grieve and grow.

There's something I call critical mass. When you are only focused on your trauma, that's what dominates your entire being. It takes up all the oxygen so there's no space left for conjuring and dreaming. But if you take baby steps, creating small encounters and new experiences, they become like seeds in the earth. They sprout as you feed them, and eventually your triumphs can outweigh your grief and disappointments.

HONOR, REMEMBER, BUT DON'T LINGER

Social media has its challenges, but it also can be a vital tool for helping people find support and voice their pain. Omari Maynard encourages other grieving fathers to reach out to him through Instagram. Following the social media feeds of others who have become mental health champions can help those who are grieving feel less alone.

Rituals can also help you to move forward. It could be comforting to speak to a picture of your loved one. Tell them that you will always care about and remember them, but you're learning to care for yourself as well. Let them know that their death, which still shakes you and wakes you, is also awakening in you the recognition that you deserve to continue to thrive and live.

Find ways to honor their memory and also yourself. Maybe you go to a restaurant they always wanted to try and have a good meal in their honor. Or you take a trip to a destination that they always wanted to visit. If your loved one died from suicide, acknowledge that you understand that their death was the result of their deep pain and it's taught you to focus on what's unsettled within yourself. Seek support so you can choose to live.

Actions like these don't mean you're abandoning those who've gone on. You're not pretending they weren't here or denying how much you miss them. You're acknowledging that, in death as in life, they are a partner in helping you to become who you were destined to be, to find the happiness and purpose that you were born to have. They continue to lead, to guide, and to inspire you, both with what they accomplished and what they couldn't figure out. Now you get to take the baton and run your leg of the race.

"Hope" is a word, and it is also an acronym: Hold on. Pain ends. The chain of caring and teaching and love is eternal. And that is magnificent, and so are you.

WHAT TO TAKE AWAY

* **Take off the sunglasses.** Don't hide your grief. Tears are a release and teacher, and as important an expression as laughter.
* **Consider grief counseling.** Reach out, to a mental health professional, an elder, or a friend if your grief is preventing you from engaging in life or leading you to self-harm.
* **Take action.** Take the class, save for the house, enroll in the workshop. It's never too late to work toward your dreams even if you previously had obstacles in your way.

* **Tap social media.** TikTok, Instagram, and the social media feeds of mental wellness advocates can give you another way to find community when you are grappling with grief and in need of support.
* **Honor the dead by living.** Take the trip that your lost loved one never got the chance to take. And seize the lessons offered through their life and their death to help you achieve your purpose.
* **Hold on to hope.** Pain can feel unbearable. It can come in waves. But over time with support and care, it will ease. Know that and hold on.

CHAPTER 7

Makes Me Wanna Holler

"I imagine that one of the reasons people cling to their hates so stubbornly is because they sense, once hate is gone, they will be forced to deal with pain."

—JAMES BALDWIN

I remember the night the police made me kneel on the ground, not believing I lived in my own home.

Angela was out of town, and our twins were just three years old and asleep in their beds. Around midnight I heard a noise in the backyard.

I'm a Black man from Detroit, so when I hear a noise, I head straight to the kitchen to get a knife. I'm not joking. That's how we roll. I plucked a big, sharp blade out of a kitchen drawer and prepared to walk through the house to investigate.

Then I changed my mind. Maybe it was my gut talking. Maybe it was the Holy Ghost. Whatever or whoever spoke to me, right before I crossed in front of the big bay window in our living room, I stopped and put the knife down.

Someone may have just dropped a script on the porch, I

reasoned. I was probably overreacting. There was no need to arm myself for battle.

I paused before I got to the big picture window and headed to the front door, but in the darkness, I couldn't see anything through the beveled glass. I turned off the alarm, turned the locks, and stepped outside.

"Put your arms up," a woman screamed at the top of her lungs. "Get down on the ground!"

There must have been five or six sheriff's deputies standing in front of my house. The glare of their flashlights turned them into a blur, but I could make out the shape of their uniforms, and the bulge of their guns.

I'd watched enough *Law & Order* episodes, and even appeared in a few, so I knew exactly what to do. I put my hands in the air and got down on my knees.

"Yes, ma'am," I said calmly. "Ma'am, I live here."

Suddenly another deputy spoke. She was a Black woman. She recognized me.

"Oh Lord," she said, her voice rising from a murmur to a yell. "Oh Lord. He lives here! He lives here with his wife!"

Despite her confirmation that this was indeed my house, I didn't assume I was out of the woods. I asked the first deputy if she wanted me to go inside to get my ID. Or maybe she wanted to go in with me? I can't remember if I went in alone or not, but I did eventually retrieve my driver's license. The deputies glanced at it sheepishly and then the "I'm sorry's" began.

They said something about how a neighbor thought our family was out of town. They heard a noise. They saw a light. Something, something. Whatever, whatever.

Not only were there half a dozen deputies in front of my

house, another half dozen were combing through my backyard. That was the rustling I'd heard. You could only get to the yard through our kitchen or living room, so they must have jumped the wrought iron fence.

"We didn't mean any disrespect," they said. "Sorry for the mistake, sir."

But if I'd been a white man, there's no way they would have demanded that I get down on my knees. They would have given me the benefit of the doubt. Instead, as a Black man, I had to prove I belonged there, in a high-priced neighborhood, in a beautiful house. I knew that if I'd been spotted walking in front of the bay window with that knife, those deputies probably would have shot me dead.

I also understood what happened to me wasn't unusual. When you're a Black man, there are still too many people in this country who think we continue to live in the days of Dred Scott, when the Supreme Court declared Black people had no rights a white man had to respect. Doing the simplest and most innocuous things when you're Black and male, whether it's watering a neighbor's flowers, going for a jog, or picking up iced tea and Skittles can become a matter of life and death.

Henry Louis Gates, the Harvard scholar who interviewed Angela and me for his show *Finding Your Roots*, endured an experience similar to mine back in July 2009. A white cop believed Mr. Gates was breaking into his own home and arrested him for disorderly conduct. Then, when President Barack Obama called out that policeman's stupidity, it was Obama who was put on defense, criticized for daring to speak on how ridiculous it was that a Black man got angry because he had to prove he lived in his own house.

That cop readied the handcuffs and asked questions later.

And instead of being reprimanded, he was rewarded, invited to sit down with the President of the United States and Skip Gates, the esteemed historian he'd humiliated, over a cold beer.

So. It happens.

I didn't tell my attorney about my encounter with those deputies until a week or two later.

"You could have owned that whole town by now," he said, letting me know that he was still ready to sue.

I didn't have a clear explanation for why I didn't call him about those cops. I guess, like all Black men, I had to think strategically. We'd just moved into the neighborhood. We wanted our twins to grow up in that community without enduring any more animosity than they might already face simply because of who they were. I didn't want to make waves. I wanted to move on.

That's what we so often do as Black people. We have to weigh things, to let the mud settle and the water clear, so that we can achieve our goals, so that we can stay alive. We have to figure out what to hold on to, and what to let go. Otherwise, we'd be on fire with rage all the time, and we couldn't survive.

———

As a Black boy in Detroit, I grew up in what was basically a police state.

I can't even remember when I received "the talk" from my parents, that conversation virtually every Black mother and father has to have with their children, particularly their sons, to let them know how to act when—and it's when, not if—a cop pulled them over or hassled them for walking, shopping, or simply existing inside a Black body. It just felt like I and all my friends knew from the cradle what to do. It's as if that protective instinct was instilled in us through our mother's milk.

My buddies at the all-Black school I attended on West Grand Boulevard, and my playmates on Appoline Street, understood that if a cop approached us, we were to keep our eyes on the ground. We shouldn't talk any smack. Say "Yes, sir," "No, sir," and put your arms in the air if they demanded it. We knew the "po po," as the police were colloquially and unaffectionately called, were not to be messed with or trusted.

And it wasn't just the cops we had to fear. I remember how after the 1967 riots, trigger-happy soldiers stormed the streets, ready to take out people whether or not they'd done anything wrong. They were assaulting boys and men, and some women too, inflicting the same brutality that had led people to nearly burn the city down in the first place.

I was a good kid. My parents sent me to the Boys' Club every afternoon and weekend to keep me busy and spent money they didn't really have to send me to the best schools. Yet the reality is that when your neighborhoods are overpoliced, when a little Black boy gets detention while his white playmate gets a pass, you can easily get caught up in a rigged, racist system and wind up behind bars whether you deserve to be there or not.

Black boys and men have to constantly fight not to be entrapped, either literally by a bigoted cop, or more subtly by a bigoted system. It's why incarceration touches so many Black families. Even my own.

―――――

My mother grew up in Chicago, one of the main stops for Black folks moving north and west as part of the Great Migration. Her father, Lloyd Daniels Sr., was a longshoreman, unloading freight on the docks of Lake Michigan, and he rose up the ranks to become president of the local longshoreman's union.

My aunt's husband, Harry, wanted to work on the docks too, but my grandfather wouldn't help him get a job there. The wages were decent, but the life was rough and dirty and he didn't want that for his son-in-law. Uncle Harry, however, was hardheaded and insistent. He told Granddad that if he didn't bring him into the union, he wouldn't work at all, leaving my Aunt Lois, his wife and Granddad's daughter, with no income or support.

My grandfather was stubborn too. He wouldn't budge. And so, things got much, much worse.

During those terrible Midwestern winters, Lake Michigan would freeze. Goods couldn't be unloaded, and longshoremen couldn't work. So the union president would typically go in the treasury and give the longshoremen money to tide them over until the ice thawed. It was standard practice, and it was the union members' money anyway since they paid dues. But Harry went to the authorities and told them my grandfather was stealing from the treasury rather than handing the money out. And the police believed him.

Granddad fled and was on the run for months. The police would come to my grandmother's house, rousting her and her children from their sleep, looking for him. Finally, she, my mother, Aunt Lois, and my two uncles moved to Boston, where my grandmother had grown up. Granddad meanwhile remained a fugitive until he eventually got tired of running. He turned himself in and went to prison. I don't know how long he was locked up, but I know that, to this day, my family won't say Harry's name.

I believe my grandfather is the only member of my family ever to go to jail. And unlike many other Black men, he wasn't there because he turned to crime to cope with poverty or out of mental duress. Granddad was set up, railroaded, by my uncle. But the specter of prison still hung over our family, with the anger and hurt running so deep that to this day, there's a name my relatives won't speak. That was the trauma of it all.

————————

Now that Slater and his friends are starting to drive, I am having to school him about what to do when he encounters the police.

It's not a one-time discussion. It's a conversation that I have continually with him and his friends. It has to be ongoing, so they don't get complacent. So they're always on alert.

I was recently talking with my wife about a film on the life and lynching of Emmett Till that she'd seen at a screening. Miss Mamie Till, Emmett's mother, had warned her only child to be careful. This was Chicago, she told him, but he was heading to Mississippi. And it was dangerously different. Emmett, like all children, probably said or thought, "Okay, Mom. I got it." He probably figured how bad could it be?

Of course, it could be bad in ways too painful to imagine. Emmett, a beautiful child, was tortured and murdered. Even if the situation doesn't have such a devastating ending, Black boys, and girls, are often treated completely different than their white peers. And I let not only Slater, but Bronwyn, know that they'd better understand that. If people lived by the messages in the Good Book, the world would be different. But we have to deal with the world as it is.

We've got killing after killing on tape. We've seen police officers shoot Black men sleeping in their cars. We've seen a cop kneel on a man's neck until he died. And the most punishment the majority of those officers got was time off with pay. A mob predominantly made up of white people stormed the U.S. Capitol on January 6, 2021, and many were allowed to just head back to their hotels or homes without arrest. There's not a person in this world who doesn't know that if that had been a group of Black people, blood would have run through the streets and anyone who survived would be locked up for years.

In the face of that kind of injustice, a one-time conversation with our young people wouldn't cut it. We talk to them all the time, nearly every day, about the harsh realities that they're up against.

I tell my children that I don't care how smart and popular they are, or how much tuition we pay, if it's their word against that of the police, most people are going to believe the cops. Your education, income, or social standing won't matter. And with so much more at stake in your life, mouthing off at a cop just isn't worth it.

———

Believe it or not, when I think of my own encounter with those sheriff's deputies, the fear we had of the police during my childhood in Detroit, or my grandfather going to jail for a theft he didn't commit, it doesn't take me down mentally. That's because I know who I am. My family laid a strong foundation, letting me know I was smart and talented and strong. And the work I've done on myself, with Dr. K, with my dreams, with my prayer and my Lord, has only strengthened my sense of self.

But those experiences, and the broader knowledge I have of history, do remind me how vicious this American system is toward people of color. That's why the killing of Black boys and men keeps happening. The police are trained to shoot first and ask questions later because they know they can get away with it. They can say they feared for their lives, and it's often a get out of jail free card—though they probably won't go to jail in the first place.

That's why our young people shout from the rooftops that Black Lives Matter. The fact that movement, that very phrase, has to be explained illustrates the upside-down world we are caught in.

"All lives matter," some angrily clap back. "Blue Lives Matter," say the defenders of the police.

Of course all lives should matter, but it seems that the only ones that do are those that belong to white people and folks in a uniform. Black people—Black men—are declaring that our lives matter because we have no protection from the many folks who refuse to accept that.

It took one little blond girl named Amber to get an entire system put in place to find missing children. But how many Black boys had to go missing in Atlanta before someone realized it was a crime spree, and the authorities needed to investigate? I'm not interested in debating O.J. Simpson's acquittal for his wife's murder, but if those who were so horrified by the verdict could have tried to stand in the shoes of a Black person for just one second, they'd understand why some Black people cheered O.J.'s vindication.

For hundreds of years, Black people have had to suck it up, or choke it down. A man was lynched, a child was abused, a woman was raped, and we were just supposed to deal with it. Some of us understandably lashed out with violence, but others turned to the Lord and told each other it would all work out in the hereafter. They tried to salve their grief, their terror, their rage with heaping plates of food and endless prayer. We had to stay calm, to be strategic, so we and all those we loved would live to see another day.

We've grown used to the legal system rarely ever working in our favor, and that's why a not guilty verdict, even for someone as controversial as O.J. Simpson, made some Black folks rejoice, even as it enraged many white people.

So many Black boys and Black men wind up in the pipeline to jail, a dead end that strips them of their right to vote, stains them with a mark that makes it nearly impossible to get a good job, and destroys their ability to prosper or just take care of their family. And then the cycle starts all over again, when their children grow up amid all that brokenness, victimized by the same system.

The fact that so many Black men have been able to achieve, sidestepping that fate and finding a way forward despite it, is a testament to our gifts and resilience. But constantly navigating an obstacle course can wear you out. Ducking and dodging, finding a way over and around, take a heavy toll mentally. And some brothers break from the burden.

The Whole Truth

Roughly a decade ago, on whatever day of the week you picked, one of every ten Black men in his thirties was incarcerated, according to The Sentencing Project. And more than a quarter of the youths arrested in the United States were Black children, though they made up only 16% of young people in this country.

Statistics like those have been trumpeted for decades, used as evidence by people who hunted and hated Black men and boys to justify brutalizing, surveilling, and shutting them out. It's been the reasoning for the powerful to literally corral Black men, not only in jails and prisons but in certain neighborhoods and spaces. Those lines were often invisible, yet they were as sharp as barbed wire. And if a Black man stepped past them and got arrested, hurt, or killed, then it was his fault, the hunter said, because he didn't have enough sense to stay where he belonged.

Those numbers do paint a startling picture. They also contain many riddles. Why is the incarceration rate so high? What are the roots of the violence that leads so many to jail? Why do Black boys and men endure such hostility not only at the hands of those outside their community, but also often at the hands of each other?

Black people, stereotyped and discriminated against, are more likely to be locked up because they are overpoliced, less likely to be given the benefit of the doubt for actions that are excused when done by their white peers, and disproportionately convicted for crimes they did not commit. A report released in September 2022 by the National Registry of Exonerations found that while Black Americans made up slightly less than 14% of the U.S. population, they comprised 53% of those who were exonerated. That means the chance that a Black person will be wrongly convicted of a serious offense is seven times higher than someone who is white.[*]

Knowing that you are considered a criminal no matter what you don't do is mentally exhausting. Let me also add that people of a given racial or ethnic group tend to victimize those who look like them. That means white people often attack whites. Hispanics often attack other Hispanics. And yes, Black people may disproportionately victimize other Black people.

The U.S. Department of Justice's 2018 National Crime Victimization Survey found that in 62% of violent incidents involving white victims, the offender was white. Among such incidents where the victim was Black, 70% of the offenders were also Black, and in 45% of violent incidents with a Hispanic victim, the offender was Hispanic.[†]

So we can swap out the noun in "Black on Black" crime and replace it with virtually any other ethnicity.

But we are here to help Black men heal, and that means telling the whole truth. While high incarceration reflects the injustice and racism of a biased criminal justice machine, it also

---

[*] Samuel R. Gross et al., *Race and Wrongful Convictions in the United States 2022*. National Registry of Exonerations, Sept. 2022. https://www.law.umich.edu/special/exoneration/Documents/Race%20Report%20Preview.pdf.

[†] Rachel E. Morgan and Barbara A. Oudekerk, *Criminal Victimization, 2018*. Bureau of Justice Statistics Bulletin, U.S. Department of Justice Office of Justice Programs, Sept. 2019. https://bjs.ojp.gov/content/pub/pdf/cv18.pdf.

shows that many Black men need to be transformed. Because when a Black man attacks someone who could be his son, his father, or his brother, he inflicts a particular kind of terror.

Whatever the roots of the violence, a Black man hurting another Black man is a different kind of hell because it is so confusing. As Black people, we have a whole history bleeding into the present that makes us expect that we need to be on guard in white spaces. We understand that whether we're searching for housing, trying to get a loan, or walking through a department store, we are constantly vulnerable to physical, mental, or emotional assaults. And because that mistreatment is, unfortunately, predictable, we can brace ourselves for what may be coming.

But when one Black man violates another, it's doubly hurtful because it feels so wrong. It's like when a child is abused by his parents, or a teacher takes advantage of a student. It is disorienting and terrifying when the hurt happens inside the home, inside a church, or within the space that was supposed to be safe. When Black people are being harmed by Black people, there is a disconnect because we look to each other for refuge, and yet sometimes there is threat and danger among us too.

There were likely many who felt that kind of disbelief and confusion when Tyre Nichols was beaten mercilessly by five Black Memphis police officers in January 2023, leading to his death three days later. While the reasons those cops brutalized Nichols might have been rooted in the systemic oppression and anti-Blackness that lies at the foundation of policing culture, the bottom line for many Black people who saw the distressing video was that a group of Black men beat another Black man to death, seemingly without remorse.

The reasons people hurt others can be specific and complex. But often when Black men and boys victimize those who look like them, their actions are saying that "because no one saw me, I can't see you." They're saying that because their own mirror was so distorted, they couldn't see their own value, and so they can't see the sanctity of another who looks like him. They are mimicking the very oppressor whose bias and exclusion have diminished their sense of self-esteem and self-love.

Identifying with the oppressor is an emotional guardrail that can rise within any group that's been marginalized because of race, gender, sexual identity, or religion. And that person, trying to escape who they are, or trying to prove something to the group that's in power, can be more brutal to their own than any outsider.

We also live in a culture that celebrates stepping on others to get yours, and we are navigating a political moment that glorifies cruelty. The message is: "I am only worth more if you are worth less."

So when we hear about the young Black man in Chicago, or Birmingham, or Los Angeles who shoots his brother at point-blank range, we need to ask him not only where does it hurt, but who did you see? Who were you looking at when you pulled that trigger? Did you see yourself?

When we see Black men hurting other Black men sexually, physically, or psychologically, it tells me that the perpetrator who's meting out that abuse is ultimately even more damaged than the person they harmed.

I'm not just talking about the Black man who committed a crime against his brother that landed him in jail. I'm also talking about the Black corrections officer who may demean, rough up, or sexually abuse the inmate who could be his son. I'm talking about the Black prosecutor or judge who feels no mercy and grants no grace.

That's why we have to call all Black men to the floor. We have to encourage them to talk, and then we have to listen. We need to call forward the victim, and the perpetrator, because often they are one and the same.

THE HURT THAT GOES UNSPOKEN

Although Courtney has no direct experience with it, there's something we urgently need to address as we talk about anger and violence—and that is the trauma of sexual abuse.

Whether behind bars, or outside in the broader world, sexual abuse happens so much more than many will admit. So much more often than many want to believe. About 1 in 13 boys are sexually abused in the United States, according to the CDC. But the incidence is probably far greater since stigma likely reduces the number of boys or men who report such assaults.

R. Kelly was one of the most popular R & B singers in the 1980s and '90s. But throughout his career, there were always stories. Terrible, ugly stories. About how he married the singer Aaliyah when she was just fifteen. About how he abused other young girls. About how he even held them prisoner.

I think R. Kelly is a cautionary tale in many ways. On the one hand, he is a vivid example of how much disturbing behavior people will tolerate or ignore if a person is popular or famous. Too many fans didn't want to turn off the radio or mute their favorite R. Kelly songs despite the credible accusations that trailed him for years.

I understand the inclination to circle the wagons. Black men are constantly under attack and held to different standards. Like Courtney's grandfather, countless Black boys and men have been convicted, even killed, for crimes they didn't commit. But the evidence against Kelly was strong. Too many just didn't want to see it, and there's no excuse for allowing or enabling a sexual predator to keep hurting others.

Yet Kelly's story possibly highlights another grim truth. His lawyer has said that Kelly was sexually abused when he was a child. And I believe it because so many other Black men and boys have been sexually violated. I heard about the dark sexual things Kelly did, debasing girls, controlling and holding them captive, and I thought, "This brother learned how to do those things because those things were done to him. He learned how to harm from being harmed."

That is one of the main reasons we must shatter the silence around the sexual abuse of Black boys and men. We must eradicate the shame, not only so they can recover from such a searing trauma but because when the wounds of a Black man who's been violated go untreated, there's a chance he may go on to similarly attack someone else. If there's no repair after a predator crosses such a precious, intimate boundary, the victim will often go within and destroy himself, or lash out and destroy others. R. Kelly did both.

For a man who's been sexually violated, whatever his ethnicity, there is often an additional layer of emotional damage because the message of our society is that, as a man, he should have been able to protect himself. He should have been able to stop it—or he should have died trying. So he fills up with shame, and the crime against him becomes an overwhelming, life-altering secret.

There are celebrities who have courageously stepped out of the shadows to recount their experiences. Actor and former football player Terry Crews revealed in 2017 that he was groped by a Hollywood executive. He didn't say anything at the time or strike his assaulter because he feared being sidelined professionally, or that as a large Black man, he'd be the one arrested if he fought back. Chris Gardner, whose journey from homelessness to Wall Street was chronicled in the book and film *The Pursuit of Happyness*, wrote about being sexually assaulted when he was young. The singer Kenny Lattimore has also told his truth.

In an interview with television journalist Tamron Hall, Kenny shared that he'd been the victim of sexual violence when he was a little boy.

After his appearance, he says many brothers, men he'd known for years, called to say "Me too, Kenny. Me too."

The #metoo movement that became a global phenomenon a few years ago brought into the light the rampant sexual harassment of women in the workplace and led to the banishment, and sometimes punishment, of prominent abusers like the movie producer Harvey Weinstein.

But there needs to be another movement acknowledging all those Black men who've also been touched in destructive, dehumanizing ways, yet haven't gotten the support they need. Those violations have to be named so those of you who've been victimized and now struggle in your intimate relationships, those of you who grapple with depression and nightmares, those of you who hurt others in similar ways, can begin to recover.

The candor of celebrities like Terry Crews, Kenny Lattimore, and Chris Gardner is notable because the culture of hypermasculinity and its toxic ideas about what it is to be a man have made it especially difficult for Black men to speak out about being abused in such an intimate way.

There are different responses depending on the gender of the abuser. When an older woman assaults a younger man, movies and music often paint the attack as an act of seduction instead of a terrible violation. It's something he's told he should boast about and be proud of. Too many refuse to call the assault the crime that it is, or to recognize the devastating consequences it can have on that boy or young man for a lifetime.

Meanwhile, there is a starkly different reaction if the abuser is male. Unfortunately, there is still a hostility in much of our society, and particularly in the Black community, to sex between those who share the same gender. Among Black folks, religious belief and a fierce adherence to antiquated notions of manhood lead many to reject even men who are involved in loving same-sex relationships. So, if you are a man who is sexually assaulted by another man, you may receive little empathy, and your trauma is amplified. You may fear that if others were to find out what happened to you, they'd label you weak. You may not be gay, but you may still worry others will assume that you are. You may be afraid if others know that another man assaulted you, they will question your manhood.

Sexual abuse is violence, plain and simple, whoever the perpetrator. The crime says nothing about the victim, but everything about the assailant, who is too often acting out his or her own trauma by hurting someone else.

LIKE AN EARTHQUAKE

Sexual abuse ripples like an earthquake, destroying your sense of personal safety, and potentially impacting the way you love and interact with others. If you have been assaulted, you may not actively abuse someone else. But you may struggle with sexual intimacy. You may have trouble committing or being faithful within a relationship. You may take on multiple sexual partners to prove your masculinity or to dull your pain.

And so, as with so many forms of trauma, the first step toward recovery is to find someone who can hold your story. That doesn't mean the person you confide in needs to try to fix the situation. It means that they safely and simply listen.

It's best if that person is a trained clinician. Even if you're generally reluctant about the possibility of therapy, it's particularly important to seek out a professional who specializes in treating men who've been sexually abused and, if possible, one who focuses on working with Black men. Survivors of sexual violence are especially vulnerable given their trauma and the stigma that surrounds such crimes. Because, unfortunately, there are predators who may try to exploit and take advantage, a trained medical professional is the safest source of support.

So many Black men who've been sexually molested don't see themselves as credible. If you were abused, you might think, I shouldn't have roughhoused with that guy. Perhaps I shouldn't have flirted. Finding a person who can be a safe sounding board, someone who can validate your experience, letting you know that nothing you did could have justified such violence or abuse, can help you move forward on the path to healing.

We who are parents can also make sure our children are aware of the dangers they may face. Like Courtney with his children, most Black parents already have "the talk" about police with their kids. It's a conversation that's hard but necessary. It's important to realize that there are other topics that need to be discussed as well. For instance, parents and elders need to speak to our young men about how it feels to even need a talk about police and their possible brutality in the first place. Along with the admonition to keep their hands on the steering wheel or in plain sight, elicit from them what their experiences have been. Talk to them about the unfairness of it all, and how it feels for them to have to navigate such treacherous terrain.

We also need to talk to young men, as well as young women, about the sanctity of their bodies. It is important to constantly reiterate that no one is supposed to touch them without their permission, or in any way that makes them uncomfortable. If that happens, they shouldn't feel embarrassed. Come home to you, or go to anyone that they trust, and talk about what happened so they can get the help they need and action can be taken so the perpetrator doesn't hurt them, or anyone else, again.

SUPPORT BLACK MEN AND BOYS IN THE MOMENT

The deep trauma of Black boys and men, who have been sexually abused, who have been incarcerated, who have been weighed down by the crushing burdens of discrimination, fear, or poverty, requires an intervention. We have to bring mental health help to them right where they are.

The world knows how to do it. During the pandemic, governors and mayors and health officials had to figure out how to get vaccinations at no charge to a huge population. Shots were delivered in tents and drive-throughs. If you didn't have a car or bus fare, community officials offered rides to get folks to their appointments.

A similar approach can be used to support Black men and boys. We can bring them emotional and mental health support when their distress is most urgent, in authentic, grassroot ways. That can be in the barber's chair. That can be in the community center. And it can also be in the midst of moments that are volatile, like in the heat of a basketball game, or on the street.

There are violence intervention groups in many cities across the country that are trying to stem gang violence. These so-called violence interrupters, who step in to douse anger and prevent conflicts from escalating among young Black men, have taken action from Jackson, Mississippi, to Chicago and New York City. But they need support. It is highly stressful to be constantly drawn into dangerous situations where you feel a life-and-death responsibility. And if someone ends up hurt or killed despite your efforts, it can take an even heavier toll on the mediator's emotional health.

Though some experts are uncertain how effective these efforts are, they are deserving of greater research, as well as funding and training for the initiatives that are already under way. And mental health resources are essential, not only for the young men the interventions are aimed at saving but for the men who are trying to stop the violence.

We also can't just focus on the streets. Rage, fear, and the often untreated anxiety and depression afflicting so many Black boys and men can lead to explosive conflicts erupting in spaces ranging from the playground to the basketball court.

In *Playing with Anger*, Dr. Howard Stevenson looks at the relationship between basketball and anger.* What if we stepped up to young men on the court, taking the pressure down in those moments when a fight is about to break out on the sidelines or beneath the hoop? It might enrage some fans who want the game to go on, but such an intervention might keep someone from getting physically hurt while beginning to get at the underlying emotional pain that likely sparked the confrontation in the first place.

So often, even with professional athletes, a fouled ball or a misguided elbow is a flashpoint, but it's not really about the competition. It's about the shame of missing a shot. It's about feeling insecure and needing to save face. It's about buying into limited ideals about masculinity and feeling you need to swagger and retaliate. But if someone steps in with expertise and care, instead of balling up his fists, he may instead learn how to manage uncomfortable emotions while handling his aggression.

All of us, Black boys and men and those who love them, can help create those opportunities. We can create our own Marshall Plan. Just as religious institutions, Black Greek

---

* Howard C. Stevenson (ed.), *Playing with Anger: Teaching Coping Skills to African American Boys Through Athletics and Culture*. Praeger, 2003.

letter organizations, and various community groups rally to register people to vote, they can do similar outreach for the purpose of improving our community's mental health.

Hotlines can be set up. Conflict mediators can be on call. While mental health professionals can't be on-site everywhere, therapists and social workers can be enlisted to train everyday folks on what to do to cool down heated moments. If enough parents, teachers, and neighbors become aware that there is more behind someone "popping off" than their simply being hotheaded or "having an attitude," and they also have a tool kit they can tap for resources that can intervene, we can keep regretful incidents from happening and also launch a broader mental health conversation.

Black people and our allies are beginning to collectively develop lifesaving strategies that I believe will create an ever-growing number of spaces and platforms where Black men are not just invited in but truly feel at home to explore themselves. Then, when they see themselves reflected in their brothers, the response will most often be, "I understand. And I'm here to help."

WHAT TO TAKE AWAY

* **Sexual abuse is not your fault.** It may be among the most devastating violations, but your hurt is not to be shamed. Find a teacher, a social worker, or another trusted friend or acquaintance to talk to about what happened. And consider seeking counseling.
* **Expand the talk.** Don't just tell Black boys how to behave when they encounter the police. Ask them how it feels to have to have such a conversation in

the first place. Ask them their feelings about navigating such injustice. And let them know that no one is ever supposed to touch them in a way that makes them uncomfortable.

* **Meet Black men in the moment.** We can try to defuse moments of tension, whether they're on a street corner or on a basketball court, before they grow out of control. Not only might it prevent someone from getting physically hurt, but it may lead those involved to begin a deeper exploration of the self-doubt and insecurities that sparked the conflict in the first place.

* **It's not helpful to say calm down.** Ask the important question, please tell me more . . . Let black boys and men know that "I see you, and I hear your pain." Don't shut them down, safely make space for them to express their heart's truth.

CHAPTER 8

Paying It Forward

"The Greatness of a man is not how much wealth he acquires, but in his integrity and his ability to affect those around him positively."

—BOB MARLEY

Not only did my mother stay in our family home after my father's suicide, she spent the next thirty years building a new life.

When I arrived in Detroit that day in 1990, my mother was not only grieving, she felt helpless. She was a smart woman. She'd always worked. But Dad handled everything, from paying the bills to maintaining the family car.

I found Mommy puddled up on the floor crying in front of a silent TV. "I don't even know how to work the VCR," she said quietly.

But she learned.

In addition to seeing a therapist to help her deal with my dad's death, my mother leaped into the daily tasks she now had to juggle on her own. She filled in her social calendar, spending time with relatives and friends.

And when she retired after decades working as a librarian, she gave to others ferociously. She continued to return to the library where she'd worked, teaching children how to read just like she'd taught Cecilie and me. She volunteered at a local soup kitchen and at the Detroit Institute of Arts. And she drove 20 miles to work out at her gym four times a week.

She was giving her children a master class in how you can start again after a hard ending, and not just go through the motions, but really relish living. A key part of that was giving to others, passing along caring, and wisdom and love.

I watched her with awe. And then, just as she taught me how to read, and to persevere, I had to embrace her sense of duty and purpose when Mom got ill.

At first, we weren't sure what was going on. Mom would speak, and one syllable would slide into another, or a word would come out muffled. We chalked it up to her dentures or thought maybe we just didn't hear her right. It took 7-year-old Slater to make us acknowledge what we'd all been noticing but maybe didn't want to see.

"Nana," he said one day while she was visiting us in California, "why do you talk funny?"

Angela and I chuckled a little bit, but then we had to admit that, yes, we'd also noticed Mom wasn't speaking as clearly as she used to. So, when she flew back to Detroit, I went, too, and accompanied her to an appointment we made with her doctor. It was the first of many.

We saw her primary care physician. Then a neurologist, and then another. No one could figure out what was wrong. Finally, a full year later, we got an appointment with Dr. Richard Lewis, who taught at Wayne State University. And at last, we got a diagnosis.

I now know why so many doctors couldn't come up with a definitive answer. Mom had a diagnosis that they probably didn't want to give. It was amyotrophic lateral sclerosis, also known as ALS, or Lou Gehrig's disease, named for the legendary baseball player who was crippled by it. It's a progressive illness that weakens your muscles as it attacks cells in your brain and spine. Medication and physical therapy might temper it, but there is no cure.

Now we all had to figure out how to go forward.

Several years earlier, when the twins were babies, Angela had asked Mom to come live with us. She was as much Angela's mother as she was mine and Cecilie's, so Angela loved having her close and we figured that, instead of hiring a nanny, it would be great if the kids could be in the care of their grandmother. Mom wasn't ready to make a move, though, in part because my nephew, Cecilie's son Caleb James, just wasn't having it.

I remember when Slater and Bronwyn were born and Mom was preparing to come meet them for the first time. "Why does she have to go out there?" Caleb asked when he was about three or four. "She don't even know them!"

Because Cecilie couldn't always head to California and we couldn't always pick up and go to Detroit, we literally tussled every year over who would have Mom for the holidays. And though she visited often, the bottom line was that Mom had a vibrant life back in Detroit that she didn't want to leave. Her book club met regularly, and she drove twenty miles each way to a sports club right by General Motors' headquarters to work out four times a week.

Four. Times. A week. She was a woman in her seventies, hitting the weights and the StairMaster so hard that when I'd go with her, other gym members would stop me.

"Mr. Courtney, your mother is something else!" someone would say. Mom would tell them to hush, and brush them aside, but she'd smile. And I'd beam with pride. She was beloved.

So, since Mom was firmly rooted in Detroit and not moving to Los Angeles, Angela and I went ahead and hired a nanny. The first person we hired tried to renegotiate the salary we'd agreed upon while she was departing from our interview with her. When I asked her why, she hemmed and hawed, but I'd heard enough. I told her this wasn't going to work out, and so bye-bye. To find someone new, I headed to our church, West Angeles COGIC, the next day. They had a children's ministry, and there were always people offering to help out their fellow churchgoers. Sure enough, when I checked the volunteer list, I found the name of the woman who would save us—Terrilyn.

We called her TT. She was a professional nanny who was raising her own son by herself. Because she supported her family by caring for other people's children, she put in place a whole routine and village to help raise that young man. She had a footstool by the refrigerator so that he could reach the cabinets or the top shelves of the refrigerator to get his milk and cereal. And then, after she enrolled him in a Catholic school across town that he needed to take public transportation to get to, she lined up a whole bunch of guardians to keep watch all along the journey, including the bus drivers. Mr. Jones was behind the wheel of the first bus he'd take. Then, Mr. Waters, another driver, would carry TT's son on the last leg of his trip.

TT brought that same kind of precision and discipline to our home, so Bronwyn and Slater were in order. She had them from the time they were six months until they were ten years old. And you know how children fall in love with the person who feeds and soothes them. They adored her. If Angela and I both had to be out of town and leave the twins with TT, we didn't worry for a moment because she raised her son the same way we were raising our children. Still, she didn't get confused. She was well aware that these were our kids and she made sure she pointed them back to us when we got home. She was an invaluable part of our family.

But Angela never stopped thinking our children's Nana should eventually come live with us. We had plenty of space, the weather was mild, and Caleb was getting older. So, in 2013, Mom reluctantly agreed. She was already starting to pack when we got the ALS diagnosis. Now, her coming to be with us was more important than ever. Yet we had no idea what type of odyssey we were about to embark upon, the twists and turns we'd all have to navigate, sometimes blindly, for the next four years.

TT remained with us, and that was a serious blessing because after Mom got to California, she deteriorated rapidly. She was still able to walk, but because ALS affects all things muscular, her breathing eventually became labored. Then she began to have trouble swallowing. Mom, barely able to drink a milk-shake, started losing weight. Finally, her doctors suggested we put in a feeding tube.

"It's a twenty-minute procedure, so no big deal," they told me and Cecilie, who helped my mother move from Michigan. Mom wouldn't even have to stay in the hospital overnight.

But when the day came, the doctors had trouble putting the tube in. They tried three times and just couldn't do it. And then something else clearly went wrong. Mom had walked into the doctor's office that morning on her own, but was so weak after the procedure that we had to bring her home in a wheelchair. She still could barely eat and now she was also in serious pain. We took her back to the hospital, and there we learned that during the procedure, the doctor had nicked her.

I nearly lost my mind. He nicked her? It was supposed to be a simple procedure. We wanted to be sure. But the damage was done. Mom came home in that wheelchair. And she never walked again.

Two or three times, we had to take Mom to the emergency room, where they'd intubate her since she still struggled to eat and would often choke. Finally, they said they couldn't keep doing it because it was hurting her throat. We had to consider putting in a trach.

All these decisions were descending upon us so fast and furiously, we often couldn't think straight. Mom didn't want the trach, but we really didn't have a choice. Then, breathing became so difficult, she had to go on a ventilator. At first she was still able to take some breaths on her own, but before long, the machine had to catch all the air for her.

We never considered putting Mom in a nursing home. I know some people don't have any other option, but we felt it was out of the question. However, we could no longer handle what was going on with Mom on our own. We had to get her round-the-clock nursing care.

We wound up with a rotating team of five nurses. We also hired a physical therapist, who worked with Mom so that her hands and feet didn't start to atrophy as her muscles withered. Every two weeks, we had a manicurist come to the house to do her nails, and an acupuncturist popped in every other Sunday. And Miss Katie, the lady who did Bronwyn's hair, also styled my mother's locs.

She had a routine. We had a routine. We all adjusted to our new rhythm.

Cecilie's home and job were thousands of miles from California so she couldn't always be with us. But every afternoon, at 4:30 p.m. sharp Pacific Standard Time, she'd call, and we'd set up an iPad on the mantlepiece in front of Mom so the three of us could spend time together.

We'd be cracking up, replicating the rituals of our family that had been there when we were kids, when mom was healthy, when our father was here. We'd watch NBC news with Lester Holt, and Cecilie and I would call him "No Lip Lester" (or was it "One Lip Lester"?) because his lips never seemed to move. I respect the brother, so it was all in good fun. Fun was the goal. We were trying to lighten the mood.

Mom would just lie there rolling her eyes, but I know she enjoyed just being able to listen to her children talk even though we were chatting about literally nothing. We found beauty in the smallest and simplest of things.

Before long, Mom could only blink her eyes and move her left thumb well enough to hit the bell to summon someone to give her what she needed. That bell was a problem, technically funky, not ringing like it was supposed to. We also had problems with a device we bought that was supposed to speak for Mom. It was similar to what the physicist Steven Hawking used, but we couldn't get that thing to work most of the time. So we had to improvise. We broke the alphabet down into clusters of letters on a board. "ABCDE" for instance would be the first quadrant. "FGHIJ" would be the second. Mom would blink her eyes a certain number of times to spell out a word. But obviously that was very slow and tedious. It was incredibly frustrating for her to communicate.

Mom was in that nearly paralyzed state for two years. Blinking her words, relying on a ventilator, getting nutrition through a trach. Her decline was swift after that incompetent doctor nicked her trying to put in a feeding tube. And her physical condition was a constant, stark reminder of all that so many of us take for granted. The muscles and systems, the neurons and synapses. They work in such mystical synchronicity that we assume that it will always be that way. But when the systems fail, and we and our doctors try to re-create what God does, we can't do it.

Try to make your brain work by your own will, or to autofocus your eyes so you can see what's in front of you and whatever objects are behind it on your own. You can't. We had a good friend who had a series of strokes, and just trying to hold on to the memory of what he'd done ten minutes before was impossible. He could recall what we talked about when we first met twenty-five years ago. But ask what he had for breakfast that morning, or why he'd just entered the room, and he drew a blank. It was devastating.

So many of us take so much for granted.

We adjusted to our new normal, the nurses and neurologists, the frequent doctor visits and all the machines. Bronwyn and Slater were part of the mix too. Our time with Cecilie ended at 6:00 p.m. Then, before Mom's last nurse left for the day, we'd hoist her into a Hoyer lift and gently lay her down in her bed. Mom never wanted her grandchildren to see that whole process. But once that was done, we'd call them into her bedroom and they'd tell her all about their day. Then they'd leave to have dinner, and do their homework, coming back a couple hours later to kiss her good night.

All of us, Slater and Bronwyn too, were learning how life was all about pivoting, all about finding the laughter and the light, so you don't lose your mind. It's about grabbing every bit of joy you can find as you care for those you love and do for them like they did for you.

You do even for those who've never given you a thing. Like Mom did back in Detroit for those young children she tutored and hungry families she helped to feed. You don't offer a piece of advice, buy someone in need some groceries, or simply open a door so you can get a thank-you or applause. You do what's right because it's right. You do things for others because, whether we know each other's name or not, we are part of a global community.

We rented a Honda Odyssey van with a lift to take Mom to her frequent doctor appointments. And we bought her a motorized wheelchair. It was a whole process, and Mom's nurse, our Executive Assistant, Miss Anita, and I operated in tandem, like parts of a fine-tuned machine. When we got to the doctor's office, we even had a soundtrack. I'd crank up the volume on my phone and blast Aretha Franklin singing "Dr. Feelgood." We'd walk into that doctor's office, where there was never good news, like we were heavyweight champions bounding gleefully into the arena.

It all took patience. Patience I'd learned through therapy. Patience I'd learned through faith. I'd also learned to find peace amid sorrow from my experience loving Bottom.

Bottom was the beautiful dog I owned while I performed in *Six Degrees*. He was named for a central character in Shakespeare's *A Midsummer Night's Dream*.

Bottom was so attached to my heart that he was often a character in the dreams that I relayed to Dr. K, and he was the companion I walked before I raced back to my apartment to get my rest.

At one point he'd gotten sick, and a Good Samaritan—a nurse I'd never met before and would never see again—offered to take a sample of his blood and send it to a vet she knew. We found out that Bottom was slowly being poisoned by the food he was eating and likely would have died in just a few weeks if that nurse hadn't intervened. Again, God had put the right person in my path. Nothing is random. The nurse put me in touch with the upstate NY holistic vet for whom I had been looking for two years. (Dr. Marty Goldstein). I changed Bottom's diet, and his fur, which had grown patchy and matted, grew back thick, shining like silk.

But the day came when he got sick again and this time there was no cure. Bottom's hips began to deteriorate, and he couldn't go for long walks anymore. We'd go outside, walk up the block a little bit so he could do his business, and then he'd lie down on whatever patch of grass he could make it to while I sat down on the curb. We'd be there for forty minutes or so, watching the world flow by. I'd think about life during those precious final days, appreciating my time with Bottom too much to obsess on being sad. I had to be still, finding the hope in the twilight. And I was comforted by the comfort I gave.

After Cecilie signed off from our evening calls, the kids were doing their own thing and Angela was watching one of the TV shows she loved, it was time for just Mom and me. The nurse had bathed her by then. She was in her bed, and we'd sit in her room watching TV. *Breaking Bad. Game of Thrones.* CSI Miami. We'd be into it, watching an episode, or two, or three.

Mom would want to keep watching, but when it got close to midnight, I'd tell her I had to get to bed.

"I've got to work in the morning, Mommy," I'd say. "But you watch another episode." She'd blink her eyes no. I'd turn off whatever show we'd been watching and turn on one of the *CSIs*. And she'd watch as she and her nurse fell into their nighttime routine.

When Mom eventually went into hospice, and the time finally came when we had to say "See you soon," I asked everyone to give the room to my sister, who'd come to be with us during Mom's final days, and me.

"I've got the show cued up, Mommy," I said, grabbing the remote. "You ready to watch? Or if you're tired, we can save it for tomorrow." I just wanted one more night with her. Just one more night.

But there wouldn't be a tomorrow. Mom's eyes told us so. She blinked and it was clear what she was saying. "Baby, I've seen everything I want to see. I've got to go."

The ventilator. The intubating. The hole that enabled her to eat. She'd had enough. She was tired of all the poking and prodding. She'd taken all of that to be here for me and Cecilie and Angela and the grandbabies. And now she was making a choice for herself.

There's a finite number of breaths we take on this earth, and I saw my mother take her last. When she left this world, I was blessed to be right there, whispering in her ear.

"It's okay," I told her. "If you're tired and ready, let go."

There's something about seeing death happen that can anchor you. It can make you decide, *I'm not messing around. I ain't got time.*

When my mom became a widow, she got busy. When she retired, she got even busier. She taught all of us who loved her how to live, how to move on, how to transition. She taught us that once you leave your job, you're supposed to fill your days with even more activities because you don't have any excuse now not to do all you need and want and love to do. You have to find new passions to fuel you, because eventually the career ends, your children grow up, but the world keeps turning.

We had Mom's homegoing back in Detroit, and during the days we were there, I discovered that there was nowhere you could go in that city that folks didn't know Miss Leslie. Everybody came to her to tell them their problems. She'd been quietly and steadily doing and helping and teaching folks all over our community her entire life. She was the resident griot and it seemed everybody in town knew that except her own children.

So many people came to her service, we couldn't fit them all in the church. That's how much love she earned by paying her own love forward. And I understood more clearly than ever before that that was what life is about.

I remember when I was in my late thirties, and I was complaining to my godly counselor, Dr. Frank Little, about some responsibilities I had. He looked at me.

"Courtney, you've played for thirty-seven years. Ain't that enough? It's time to focus on other people. That's the next phase. That's the evolution of life, to grow up and to give back."

I truly believe that working with Dr. K enabled me to better care for Bottom. I believe being with Bottom made me more selfless for my wife, Angela. Caring and doing for Angela and our children got me ready for the responsibilities and sacrifices that would be required to take care of my mother.

You have to be of service, to your family, to your community. It can be a juggling act, and sometimes some of the balls fall or the plates crash to the floor. But if you keep at it, if you recognize the importance of it, you get better at all the balancing.

I know how overwhelming life can be. But when we look out for one another and speak honestly to others about whatever we're going through, we gain companions on this sometimes daunting journey. They may be able to help us see that whatever it is we're going through isn't as bad as it first seemed. Or maybe it is, but it will pass. We can gain clarity. And then we can ask ourselves as we wrestle with a tough situation, "What you gon' do about it? What's the plan?"

When you do for others, you form connection. And then, no matter how bad the storm, you're anchored like a buoy to the bottom of the sea, and you can ride the waves. You're still going to deal with stuff. It may still be painful and frightening. But you know that you have a foundation, rooting you to the world.

I spent four years caring for my mother, watching her strong spirit remain even as her body broke apart. I've seen my teenage twins wrestle with their own emotional struggles, forcing me to accept that while we hate to see our children suffer, they can't avoid ditches and gulfs that come with living. I've had to deal with the reality that while I am a great actor, I might never be a global superstar. And I'm at peace with all of it, because I'm anchored.

I began to learn in the years that I spent with Dr. K journaling and dreaming that my being here in this life is not about me. It's about me taking all I know, all I have, and helping somebody else. And that grounds me. I know that who I am is not where I live. I'm not how much money I make, or what awards I receive. My gratification comes from Angela and I seeing our children grow into respectful, kind, young adults, and knowing that I had a hand in that. My gratification comes from hearing that a young man sought mental health support after hearing me share my own emotional trials. I am grateful when I see that my experiences, my truth, are helping someone else hold on, get up, and strut on.

That's why I speak about and attend events for the Boys & Girls Clubs, which did so much for me in my childhood and helped pave my way to Country Day. It's why I talk to prospective students applying to Harvard and, along with Angela, offer encouragement to young performers who want to do what we do.

And it's why I keep on writing and speaking about my mental health journey, the losses I've experienced, the therapy that helped me through, so my brothers can realize that, no, they are not crazy, no, they are not alone, and there are anchors to grab on to if they are willing to reach for them. It's why I talk about the epidemic of suicide among our young Black men, and the experiences I personally had with my godson as well as my father.

I want to let those in so much emotional pain that they're contemplating taking their own lives know that we've all had moments of utter despair. But if they just hold on, if they go to a therapist, see a doctor about medication, talk to a friend, call up their religious leader, they can get through it. And then when they meet that romantic partner they dreamed of, get that job they wanted, or just have the opportunity to sit and gaze at one more sunset, they will be so glad they did.

There's More to Life

When you reach out to someone else, you never know what that will do. You may save his life or your own. Or you may help him discover the life he was meant to live.

I once interviewed the artist J. Ivy. He's a significant, impactful poet whose fingerprints are all over the pop culture landscape. He's worked with some of the most popular hip hop artists of our time. He even gave the singer and activist John Legend his name.

J. was recording with Jay-Z and Kanye West when someone in the studio played him some music created by a singer named John Stevens. When J. and John met, J. told him that his sound reminded him of the old-school artists his parents used to play. He told him that he sounded like one of the musical legends.

"Yeah," he repeated. "You're John Legend."

Others began to echo J., and eventually John Stevens took the hint, and changed his name to a moniker that proclaimed his brilliance.

J. and I talked about the necessity for Black men to nurture themselves and to feel entitled to self-care. We discussed how self-care was still a foreign concept to many, but it was becoming more familiar as men like J. made a point of carving out spaces to talk about how tending to their own emotional needs made them better partners, artists, fathers, and members of the community.

I asked him what was his wake-up moment? What called him more fully into being who he was born to be? It turns out that he was a teenager when he discovered that what he was telling himself about himself was all wrong. It was a tenth-grade English teacher in Chicago whose encouragement enabled him to flip the script.

Her name was Miss Paula Argue, and yes, the irony of her name wasn't lost on her students. They'd joke that you didn't argue with Miss Argue. One day, she gave everyone an assignment: Write a poem.

J. figured he'd just throw some words down on paper about clouds so he could hurry up, finish, and get back outside to hang with his boys. He showed up the next day with his short sonnet about the sky, prepared to just hand the piece in when Miss Argue hit him and the other students with a surprise. She wanted everyone to stand in front of the class and recite what they'd written.

J. just knew that was going to be a disaster. Here he was a cool young guy who'd thrown together a poem about clouds. How was he going to get up in front of everyone and read that? But you didn't argue with Miss Argue. So J. read the poem. He got a standing ovation.

It was the first time J. realized he had a gift. He also got an A along with an invitation. Miss Argue wanted him to recite his poetry in a talent show.

He was not on board. J. was a shy kid, he said, whose parents had gotten divorced, an event that had a heavy impact on him. But just as Ms. Argue affirmed his talent with a top grade, she wanted to push him further. She made it a mandatory class assignment to participate in the talent show. The response J. received when he recited his words validated his talent even more.

He realized that he had something. He was both a shy child of divorce, and a great writer and performer. His mother also recognized his writing talent and J. went on to attend Illinois State University, rhyming his truth from stages around Chicago to HBO's Def Poetry. Since then, his writing and collaborations have been recognized and honored by the Peabody and NAACP Image Awards. He's successfully gotten the Grammys to break poetry out into a separate category all its own.

That's the power of passing it on, of giving praise and encouragement to others, of telling Black boys and men that you see their talents as well as their fears. The script in J.'s head about what he couldn't do got a rewrite and helped him become the man he was meant to be—a gifted artist helping others to express their creativity and share broad truths about identity, about Blackness, and whatever else they want to give voice to.

Who serves that purpose in your life, motivating you, shouting out gifts that you may not have known you had? Think about it, and if you can't come up with someone, make it a goal to start surrounding yourself with people who see you and want to lift you up.

How many Black men have been lost because they didn't have anyone to affirm the gifts that only they could give? I'm not saying that everyone is going to be J. Ivy, working with Jay-Z, or Kenneth Chenault, the former CEO of American Express. But they don't have to be. Because whatever each of us brings to the table is uniquely ours. If you didn't have a singular contribution to make, you wouldn't be here. Period.

That's why the dichotomy of being either invisible or seen as a violent, unworthy caricature, is so devastating. It can stop exploration of yourself before it even begins. This leaves too many Black men veering down a dangerous path, thinking they are in control when there are others who care nothing about them who are really behind the wheel.

GIVE GOOD CARE

Mentoring, caregiving, and friendship can fill the lives of Black men, and those who love them, with a purpose that is mentally fortifying.

Looking after a loved one, like Courtney and his family tenderly did for his mother after her ALS diagnosis, is perhaps the most obvious form of caregiving. I too made this herculean commitment to care for my mother until her death in May 2020. But caregiving is just as critical for those in your life who are struggling emotionally, whether that's asking them where it hurts, checking in with them from time to time, or helping them find additional support if they need it so they don't stay stuck in their past and their pain.

Being a mentor is another way to pass along care. You can take under your wing the young man who shovels your snow for a few dollars in the winter, who serves you coffee at the local Starbucks, or who sits in the back of the math class that you teach.

You can ask him what he is interested in. If you see him doodling and notice the beauty of the lines, talk about his potential as an artist. Is he naturally funny? Does he enjoy science fiction? Reaching out helps others to open up, not only about their struggles but also about their dreams. You can help them imagine their future, and perhaps help them decide to alter their path by reshaping their present.

And of course, some of the greatest care you can give to another is through friendship. Just being that person with whom a young man feels he can share his longings, his loves, and his insecurities can give solace and comfort.

That doesn't mean taking on more than you can bear. If a friend is causing you distress, you may want to tell him that you may not be the best support for him in this moment, but you are open to finding other pillars that can help hold him up. However, being a friend does sometimes entail dealing with your own discomfort, and so if it's not too heavy a burden, be there to listen. And hopefully when you are in need, they will return the favor.

GET IN PEOPLE'S BUSINESS

We can help each other out in the most fleeting of encounters, even if we have never met before and will never meet again. With so much at stake, it's important to set aside the adage that we need to stay out of other folks' business and recognize that we all have a stake in each other and so we may need to get involved if someone's emotional frame of mind is hindering their potential, fueling self-destructive behavior, or leading them to possibly hurt others.

Perhaps this idea is unpopular, as these days, we're often advised to mind our own business. Of course, we must also trust our intuition, sizing up the situation so that we don't jeopardize ourselves emotionally or physically. And it's definitely not healthy to focus on other people's business as a way of avoiding your own emotional challenges and issues.

When you're checking in with a loved one or a stranger about an emotional episode, it can be like stepping onto an icy lake. You have to step gently, careful not to push too hard so you don't endanger yourself or anyone else. But at the very least, you can let them know you can relate to what they're going through and that you care.

It's like when you see a father at the store, growing impatient with his young son. Yes, you can ignore it, figuring it's not your business. But if we are indeed our brother's and sister's keeper, the more helpful move might be to figure out how you can mirror that stranger who's clearly at his wit's end.

Maybe you just try to catch his eye and offer a nod and a smile. Maybe you let the moment pass, head to the line he's standing in, and simply say, "I don't know about you, but I know today's a hard day for me."

Perhaps he'll respond, saying how frustrating it is that these kids want everything, like money grows on trees. Maybe he'll crack a smile, or make a joke.

He might chuckle. He might calm down. Maybe when he gets back to the car, he'll start kidding around with his son, relieving the tension that built between them in the supermarket.

Your tiny action can spark a series of other, positive reactions. Speaking to that man, in that moment, lets him know I see you and I don't blame you. Let's pause. Let's exhale. There's no telling what a minute of compassion can do.

To continue this point, as we try to pass along love and care, we may also need to question what traditions and actions we've been passing on that need to stop. For all the good groups like fraternities, sports teams, or school clubs do, they have been known to engage in initiation practices that are dehumanizing, like hazing, paddling, and punching— or worse, in the case of street gang organizations.

I ask members of those organizations to wake up, and ask themselves who told you that beating or humiliating someone who is trying to become your brother was a good idea?

We talk about how we want this country to own what it has done to Black and brown and indigenous people. We rightly lambast them for trying to rewrite or erase history, banning literature and literally removing books from library shelves. But it is also important for Black men who band together to look in the mirror and ask themselves whose narrative they are living out if and when they diminish young men who want to be a part of their community? How does putting your hands on another Black man and harming him demonstrate or lead to loyalty and connection?

There is something sadistic and pernicious in the systemic architecture of this nation, that exploits and hurts people. The audacity to tell injured people to trust and be loyal to a system that has betrayed them is obscene. It is a form of gaslighting that we find in too many facets of American life.

Unless members of these groups are willing to look at whose narrative they are playing out, including the hyper-masculine posturing that often leads to womanizing and excessive drinking, unless they are willing to honestly say out loud how those cues and codes harm Black people, and Black men in particular, and adopt a new way of initiating and being together, they are just repeating cycles of diminishment created by others who have no regard for Black lives.

If we are asking Black men who are hurting each other emotionally and physically on the street corner or on the playground to stop and take a breath before they inflict harm, if we want them to ask who they see before they hurl an insult or fire a shot, we can ask no less of the young men on college campuses, on the football team, or in the high school band who may one day be the leaders of our broader community. It will take courageous Black men to tell the truth and call out harmful traditions. It will take strength to say, I don't know when this started but I'm awake to the truth that a Black man beating or belittling another Black man is always a bad idea. It serves no purpose and has no redemption.

I SEE YOU

J. Ivy has a motto he's known for: "Dreams don't come true. They are true."

When we take the grace and love we've been given and pay it forward, wrapping Black boys and men within it, it allows them to imagine who they can be. Or they may realize they have been that awe-inspiring person all along.

Sometimes all it takes is taking the time to let them know that we see them.

I'm a jogger, and recently I was out for a run. I ran into a group of young Black men coursing through the neighborhood. Some were cruising in their cars, pumping their music, while others whizzed by me on their bikes. I believe they were all coming from and congregating around a nearby park.

We were in an upscale, mostly white neighborhood and I have no doubt that many of the residents probably weren't particularly happy to see those young men there. But it was a beautiful summer day. Everyone wanted to be outside, and so where should those young brothers be? Where should they go?

I knew that many of the passersby probably didn't see them as worthy of a greeting, of a "How are you?" or "How are you doing?"

So I made an effort to catch their attention.

"Good morning," I said to some.

"Have a nice day," I said to others.

And then I followed each of those greetings with a prayer.

"Be safe."

I wasn't just telling them to be safe on their bikes. I was saying to be safe in their bodies. I was saying, "I see you and I know you're often not seen, and if you are, people too often label you as a threat, and then that may become how you see yourself."

If that was the case, I wanted them to reimagine themselves, to see a new image in the mirror. I wanted those young beautiful brothers to know that I saw them not as strangers, not as a menace, but as the whole, gorgeous human beings that they were. I wanted them to know that I wanted them to have a wonderful day and many more splendid days ahead.

Some looked startled by my words. They seemed rattled by the recognition, surprised by the warmth.

Then, they smiled.

WHAT TO TAKE AWAY

* ✳ **Get in other folks' business.** You can let someone who is struggling know that you see them in the most stressful, but also most ordinary, of moments.
* ✳ **Change the script.** Organizations of Black men can look at their own patterns and traditions and change them if they are harmful, mirroring a narrative written to harm them.
* ✳ **Say "I see you."** Just offering a friendly greeting can be soothing and uplifting.

CHAPTER 9

Take Good Care

"If you don't love yourself, nobody will. Not only that,
you positively won't be good at loving anyone else.
Loving starts with the self."

—WAYNE DYER

As long as we live, we are going to have to struggle. There's no avoiding it. What we need is to have the tools to help us get back up, to help us remember that this, too, shall pass.

The time I spent in therapy with Dr. K, filling journals with my dreams, saved my life. They resembled my blue books in high school and college, but instead of calculus and Latin, I was reflecting on and studying myself.

But there came a time when I needed something more. I'd always believed in God and gone to church, but I didn't always feel the power of what the pastor said. And then I had a crisis that brought me home.

Romantic relationships are hard. I doubt there's any man who would disagree. Angela and I loved each other deeply. But when we first got married, we found ourselves struggling on how two become one. I didn't know how to bring us together, to get to the point where instead of each of us competing to be right, we competed to show who was the most understanding, who was the most giving, who was the most caring. I knew we had it in us. We just had to trust each other enough to tap into that all-consuming love we felt for one another and show it completely every day. Because when you don't have that trust, walls rise up, and if you're not careful, they may grow too high to overcome.

But I just didn't have the tools, the know-how, to bridge the distance widening between us. So I nitpicked instead.

"How could you be gone all day at the movies and not call?"

"You're going out with your friends *again*? I thought we would spend the evening together."

All my questions just made Angela feel bad. They made her feel judged, and guilty, and it drove her to not want to engage with me.

For one of the few times in my life, I was failing. I couldn't figure out how to help Angela, how to help me, how to help us. I was being pulled under, terrified of messing up this wonderful thing. I thought I might be having a nervous breakdown.

One night as I lay in bed, my dreams dissolved into nightmares and I was shaking uncontrollably while I slept.

Angela woke me. Then she called the doctor.

The next thing I knew, Angela was pushing me into the car and jumping behind the wheel. We were headed to my doctor's office. When we arrived, he talked to me a bit. Or at least he tried to. But I wasn't very coherent. I couldn't stop the tears. I didn't know what was happening. I was getting scared.

Gulping for air, trying to calm myself, I overheard Angela and our amazing doctor, Dr. William Young, whispering outside the examination room. I caught a few words.

"Breakdown."

"Psychiatrist."

"Hospital."

Then, I heard something else.

"Do you hear me now?"

It was a voice inside my head. Only it was more than that. The voice was reverberating through my whole body.

"Are you ready?"

The voice was loud, insistent. I recognized it. It was holy.

I can't explain it, but I immediately understood what was being asked of me, like a little boy can catch the subtext of his daddy's words just by his tone. God was telling me I had to prepare for all that was coming, the good, the bad, and the in-between. I had to get ready for the jubilation I would feel raising my two precious children, and the heartache of caring for my ailing mother. I needed to prepare for the peaks of my professional success and develop the resilience required to weather the grief that would come as I continued to lose people I admired and loved.

You have to listen, the voice said. That's how you'll learn to navigate marriage with Angela. If you can't listen and learn how to strengthen your bond with your wife, you sure won't be able to respond to all the other challenges that are bound to come your way. I need you to get ready to learn how to handle this world, how to listen when it's two in the morning, you're sitting at the edge of the bed with your head in your hands, and there's no one that can help you but Me.

But to be able to fully hear, to be able to distinguish God's voice from all others, I had to do the work. God was telling me he would always be there to guide me through. He'd been there all along. But I had to be open to what he was saying.

Suddenly my tears dried up. My breathing slowed. I called out to Angela.

"I'm good now," I told her quietly when she walked into the examination room. "I know what to do. Let's go home."

I'm sure she and my doctor gave each other the side-eye. But Angela did what I asked. Maybe she'd sensed something had changed. Or maybe she just believed in me. Either way, Dr. Young said if I really felt better, I should go. Angela and I headed home.

I walked straight to the bedroom, grabbed the Bible we kept on the nightstand, and read it cover to cover. When I'd finished, I started again. The next time I read it, I took notes. I read it through five times. I needed a word, and I was searching for understanding.

I began reading a chapter of the Old Testament and a chapter of the New Testament each day. I also read a chapter of Psalms and a chapter of Proverbs. It was simple to do, and it anchored my soul. Just like I'd sought the messages in my dreams, I was now seeking the messages in the Good Book. I wanted to grab every morsel of wisdom and incorporate it into my life.

I had to study. I had to listen. I had to work, because nothing comes easy, no matter how it might appear to someone standing on the outside peeking in.

Someone could look at the trajectory of my wife's career, for instance, and assume that, with her talent and beauty, the great parts came effortlessly. But she didn't just get handed roles in films like *Mission: Impossible* and *Black Panther*. She went to the Yale School of Drama. She built her résumé project by project. Michael Jordan and Tom Brady and Serena Williams weren't simply born three of the greatest athletes of all time. They had to train, they had to practice, they had to sacrifice.

It's the same with our emotional health. When I got that call telling me my father was dead, I had to learn to accept that there were things I couldn't foresee, terrible events I couldn't control. When Angela was on the verge of having me admitted to a hospital because I was breaking down, I had to pull myself back from the precipice and try to steady my mind.

What was I so afraid of? Was I ready to do the work needed to be the husband, the father, and the friend that I wanted to be?

To be that pillar for those I loved, I began to realize that I first had to care for myself. I had to discover what practices grounded me, whether it was reading a proverb or uttering a prayer. And once I figured out what gave me clarity, what slowed my breathing, and calmed my nerves, I could always reach for those anchors when I was troubled, knowing no matter how far I drifted away from the path, no matter how deep in the woods I wandered, I'd never completely lose my way.

Therapy was my first safe harbor. It meant so much to have a place where I could go once—or sometimes two or three times— a week, and unload all that was troubling me. I could interpret my dreams without ridicule or judgment. Or sometimes I could not speak at all. I didn't feel pressured to fill the silence. I didn't have to perform. I didn't have to be perfect. I could just sit there, against that pillow with the spidery design, and just be me.

When my girlfriend and I broke up a year or so after my father's death, counseling helped me to see that there was no use wallowing in the past. Yes, I knew I'd messed it up, unable to formally commit despite all she'd meant to me. But I was taking the time I needed now to work on myself, so that whenever I got another chance to be with someone I loved dearly, I would be ready to go the distance. I thought that someone might be her, open to trying again. But I later realized I'd been preparing to meet Angela. And I would need to continue doing the work to grow alongside my wife for the rest of our lifetimes.

Eventually, however, I had to work on myself without Dr. K as my constant guide. Our relationship was always supposed to be finite. Her goal was to get me to the point where I understood how I made decisions, and be in tune enough with my inner voice, to move forward on my own. I had to learn to rely on myself when I needed to figure out whether to begin or end a relationship, whether I should take or reject a role, and all the tiny decisions in between.

So, sometime in 1995, Dr. K and I decided she had taken me as far as she could. I stopped our weekly 5:00 a.m. phone sessions (I'd been in LA for a year and a half), and I stopped jotting down the pictures and thoughts that came to me in my sleep.

Therapy had gotten me to a certain point. Faith would carry me further.

———

When I was a child, I prayed every night. There were times when I prayed harder, like when I didn't feel ready for a big test or I really wanted to score in the next day's game. Other times, prayer was just part of my routine, the thing I knew I was supposed to do like taking a shower; walking Rana and Pepper, our dogs; or saying "Yes, sir" and "Yes, ma'am" to my elders. Whether or not there was a sense of urgency, prayer was a ritual that I engaged in just once a day.

But that's not the way I do it anymore. As a husband and a father, a brother and a friend, I thank God constantly. I don't have to be on my knees to do it. When I'm waiting at a red light, standing in line at the checkout counter in the grocery store, or waiting for the water to boil to make a cup of tea, I fill that pause with prayer.

I say, "Lord, thank you," when I wake up in the morning and think about how blessed I am to see another day. When I greet the woman who delivers our mail or say goodbye to an old friend, I make sure to get in a "bless you" or "amen."

When I'm in the backyard, watching the gentleman who does our landscaping engage in his beautiful work, I thank Jesus for him and the beautiful home he's enabled my family and me to have. And I offer praise whenever I see Angela, Slater, and Bronwyn walk through the front door.

I thank God so often, and in so many ways, it's more than a prayer. It's a meditation that fills me with gratitude and a sense of peace. And on those occasional mornings when I get so busy that I forget to say the Lord's name, I actually scold myself.

"Is this the first time I'm calling your name today?" I ask when I realize I've been distracted by an errand or a script. "If that's the case, I'm sorry."

Calling God's name is my way of honoring the one who has always steered me on the right path and lined it with the amazing people I've encountered along the way. When I pray, it reminds me of who I am, and whose I am. When I pray, I remember that there is somebody in the hospital waiting room right now, anxiously looking for the doctor to come in and give them some good news, and I'm just grateful that, in this particular moment, that's not my reality.

But I know it will be my reality eventually. If we live long enough, every one of us will be in that room, waiting for a glimpse of the white coat, hoping for a smile, dreading a shake of the head. We're all either in a crisis, coming out of one, or standing in that precious gap that lies in between.

Being tethered to a higher power helped me cope with the passing of Angela's mother. Knowing I was anchored kept me afloat during the four years between my mother's diagnosis of ALS and her final days in hospice. And Angela and I have been up-front with Slater and Bronwyn that they will one day have to deal with that same heartache when we leave this world. We immerse them in faith so that, when the time comes, they can withstand it.

I still get overwhelmed. And when I do, I set aside the script I'm reading or the to-do list I'm ticking through and pick up my Bible. I take the time to read it again, from Genesis 1 to Revelation 22. I take that time for myself because I am worthy of self-care. My emotional well-being is worth tending to. I can't do an acting role justice, I can't give my all to the PTA, I can't be there for a young person I'm mentoring, if I'm troubled and falling apart.

———————

It's not just reading the holy word that sets my soul at ease. When I pick up a book that teaches me about the past, that tells me how someone else struggled and persevered, I feel inspired.

Since Mom was a librarian, the love of reading was instilled in me from the time I could recognize what a book was. My room was overflowing with the adventures of Henry the Explorer, the mischief and battles of the Greek gods, and the amateur detective work of the Hardy Boys.

I also always loved history. I spent hours learning about the military missions of Napoleon and Hannibal, the beginnings of the Roman Empire, and the travels of Marco Polo. But when I started attending Country Day, heading to school early in the morning and returning home late at night, there wasn't much room for any reading beyond what was assigned by my teachers.

I'm still very busy. But I carve out the space to feed my mind because that's something just for me. I download news articles to share with my kids over the summer, when their days are less hectic, and I can quiz them on what they've read. I participate in the parents' book club at my children's school. Then I find a corner to tuck into on a Saturday morning or weekday evening, crack open a book cover, and lose myself in the musings of a great writer's mind.

I've dived into *Caste*, by Isabel Wilkerson, where I learned that the racist hierarchy in this country was so meticulous, even the Nazis marveled at its evil genius. I've made my way through Richard Rothstein's *The Color of Law*, which describes the federal government's active role in forcing Black people into dilapidated segregated communities with substandard housing and no resources.

I've read about how legendary figures nearly broke under the weight of everyday pressures, from David Blight's biography of Frederick Douglass, who struggled with his children, to Ken Burns's writings about the indomitable Eleanor Roosevelt, driven to the depths of despair over her five kids' numerous marriages, to Ron Chernow's biography of Ulysses S. Grant, the Civil War hero whose father never thought he'd amount to much.

I read like I pray—continuously. I'm always learning, because that gives me joy. And I'm nourished by learning how other people have tried and failed and tried again, pushing forward despite the obstacles in their path.

That's why I no longer sweat the small stuff. I can't say that I never get frazzled by innocuous things. I could barely remember my own name that day at the airport when I left my phone in the town car that brought me there. But mostly, when I'm sitting on the 405 Freeway in traffic and people are honking all around me; when I call customer service and have to wait on hold; when I get the green light, but before I take off, someone is racing past in a left turn; I don't dwell on it. I don't seethe or curse.

I don't let someone else's ego, or bad attitude, send my blood pressure soaring. Because as long as no one got hurt, I know it's all right. I learned through therapy how to sit and let the water clear. I've learned from years of living that there are far bigger struggles than a traffic jam that I will encounter and have to survive. And I've learned from my faith that God's got me. Always.

———

When the storms come, the question our soul asks is, "What you gon' do about it?" That's the question for all of us, the communication we get from so many messengers from the time we're born until we're out of here.

That's what my inner voice was asking when the headmaster at Country Day threatened to kick me out of school if I didn't play on the basketball team during my senior year. That was the question I had to answer when the Yale School of Drama threatened to expel me because I'd auditioned for the film *Native Son*, which was against the university's rule prohibiting students from working professionally, but had the potential to change my life. That was the confusion I had to wade through when my father killed himself and I had to figure out how to go on.

"What are you going to do, Court?"

That's also what Dr. K wanted to know. "Can you wait for the mud to settle?" she asked.

To wait for the answers, to figure out the solution, you have to be calm. And that may require strategies and rituals to help get you there. Sometimes, I still grow impatient. Sometimes I forget who and whose I am. Sometimes I grow fearful or confused. But then I know that I need a little extra loving care. Not from my wife. Not from a friend. I need a little time to take care of my own self. I need to find the quiet within me.

So I read my Bible. I walk our family dog. I go to the bookstore and peruse the shelves.

And while I no longer go to therapy, I still fiercely believe in it. I know that I can always reach out to a professional who can help me find my way out of an emotional maze. And though my journals are now stacked in a basement, I also know that if I need to get a handle on myself, I can go back and catch my dreams.

I want every one of my Black brothers to grant themselves the gift of understanding what keeps them steady, whether it's prayer to Jesus, Jehovah, or Allah; seeing a therapist; or getting together once a week with men whose experiences mirror their own. I want them to take the time to care for themselves. To carve out not only the spaces that give them relief from the strains of life, but also those that give them simple joy.

I want them to find the buoys that will keep them afloat no matter how much they flounder, offering the support they need until they can make it to safety. And I want them, once they are ashore, to feel a soft breeze, to watch the leaves fall, and just be.

Self-Care Is Nonnegotiable

You know how when you're in high school or college, you pick out your classes for the upcoming school year? In addition to the must-haves like math or literature, there are typically electives you can enroll in—art, music, sports. They're creative courses that pique your interest but are entirely optional.

Well, for Black men, self-care is not something you can choose not to do. It's required work.

You were meant to be here, or you wouldn't be, and so you have to take care of that divine being. Your soul has work for you to do, trials to hone your spirit, experiences to help you grow. And so you have to be able to discern the lessons, to understand the mission, and to hold on long enough to be able to touch the brass ring. Just like a bear stores up nourishment and energy to help survive the long cold winters, you, too, have to find ways to replenish so you can weather your difficult seasons.

It may be hard for you to prioritize your own nurturing, to make yourself a priority in a society that purposely puts you last. It might be hard for you to believe you deserve self-love in a world that goes to great lengths to ensure that you suffer.

That's why in the midst of such resistance, self-care is a revolutionary act. It's as disruptive as boycotting a business, shutting down an intersection to protest police brutality, or marching on Washington to protect voting rights, because it girds you for the battle at hand and gives you the strength to fight whatever's next. It also reminds you that life is about more than struggle and that you have a right to claim Black joy.

So what does self-care really mean? We can use a visceral analogy to break it down.

How often have you felt pressure in your bladder, the need to go to the bathroom, but before you do, you make one more phone call? You attend one more meeting or write the check to pay one more bill. Before you know it, an hour or two have passed and now you're in trouble. You have to race down the hall before you have an accident.

Self-care means learning to Pee First. You can't do your best work if you're uncomfortable, if you're under duress. Every task you take on, everyone you encounter, benefits when you are able to focus and feel at ease. The alternative is to go through the day distracted and without clarity. You can't endure or overcome, integrate or separate, transform or transcend if you don't take care of yourself first.

Not long ago, I heard an interview with Edward Enninful, the first Black man to be editor-in-chief of *British Vogue*, about his memoir, *A Visible Man*. He spoke about how he ran himself into the ground working, but a problem he had with his eyes required him to undergo surgery and to rest so his retinas could heal. Mr. Enninful talked about how much he learned in the darkness, how that respite fired up his dreams and imagination, and when he was finally able to create again, he did some of his greatest work.

He was able to replenish himself, to fill his well and come back stronger. There is a lesson in that for all of us, but most especially for other Black men. When you don't care for yourself, there is so much you can lose. You may not only sacrifice your physical health, risking disease, a heart attack, or a stroke, you may lose your ability to explore, to create, and to become your fullest, most complete self.

You may also lose those you care for, or your ability to give them your best. If Edward Enninful wasn't able to continue his work, providing a platform to a kaleidoscope of artistic talent and beauty, the world would be poorer for it. If Courtney hadn't learned to find sustenance in therapy, reading, and prayer, he would not have been able to give so much support to his ailing mother, or to continue being a ballast for his wife and children.

It's also important to understand that there is a difference between self-care and self-medicating. Of course, there's nothing wrong with drinking in moderation if your health allows it. Working out is a way to maintain your body, and for many, it's also a way to tune out noise, and to turn into yourself.

But when those actions are taken to an extreme, when you overindulge or engage to the exclusion of other activities and people, and those same activities begin to damage your body and psyche, that is a problem.

That goes for sex too.

YOU'RE NOT LIKE A SEX MACHINE

Sex is the root of creation. It is beautiful and profound. It's an intimate connection that can bring amazing pleasure and joy. Yet too often it becomes another drug, an ephemeral way to feel good for a moment, to feel powerful or to paper over poor self-esteem. Self-care must apply to your sexuality as well. You need to always remember, and to remind each other, that your bodies are precious.

Though the motivation has typically been more about control than empowerment, society has nevertheless told girls and women that they shouldn't share their bodies with any and everyone. Boys and men, however, aren't given that message, though they, too, should know from the time they are young that their bodies are also sacred.

We need to convey that truth to those whose bodies have been violated, letting them know that they are right to mourn the part of themselves that was taken. And we need to tell it to those men who abuse their own bodies by engaging in sex without intimacy.

One of the questions I pose to the young men I counsel at the Philadelphia detention center is do they really want to put their penis just anywhere?

That usually sparks howls of laughter and a lot of jokes.

"Hell yeah!" someone will shout.

"I do!" yells another.

Then, I tell them they might want to rethink that. I remind them that life can't happen without what they're putting out. Creation requires both an egg and a sperm. That makes their penis sacred, and they might want to think about where it goes.

They're not machines, I tell them. That's the lie the hunter came up with to justify treating Black men literally like breeding bulls during the time of slavery when he wasn't working them to death in the fields to enrich himself and his family. He projected onto them his own brutality. I tell those young men that the hunter said your sexual appetite was insatiable and dangerous to justify literally hunting, hanging, and castrating you for even looking at a white woman, while he raped your mothers and sisters. He said you were incapable of love and sweetness, only lust. And therefore, you weren't worthy of kindness or affection.

I want Black boys and men to recognize the multifaceted, multitalented, complex beings that they truly are. I want them to envision their full potential and to reject the hunter's story. That goes for our artists and pop stars too, who have so much influence over those who watch their movies, listen to their music, and flock to their concerts.

We've all heard the song lyrics bragging and boasting about selling dope, shooting up the spot, and having as much sex as you can stand.

Music is a form of creative expression and I understand people from all communities have long been fascinated by machismo. What I challenge is the lack of exploration about how this has become the narrative of so many raps and songs. How often does that musical narrative lead to life tragically imitating art?

That's the conversation I don't hear enough. I want the boys and men who create the music, and those who listen to it, to think about where that story came from. I want them to understand that it is a fable written for them by someone else. And when they adopt it as their own, making it seem cool or inevitable, they are crippling and damaging themselves, giving those who want to keep them down what they want.

Living out that story can lead to bringing children into the world you don't want or can't care for. It can lead to fractured relationships and feelings of abandonment and betrayal. It can trouble your mind and leave you feeling empty.

Perhaps you do not mindlessly juggle sexual partners—most men don't. But for those who do, I know that when they find a safe space, they often reveal that what they really crave is not sex, but an emotional connection. They really want to be seen and to feel valued for who they are and not the physical pleasure they can bring.

I encourage those Black men to dismantle a false identity that isn't accurate, one that was made to serve someone else's sinister purpose. When you are focused on just putting notches on your belt, you deny yourself the comfort and inner peace that can come with true intimacy. And you deserve that. Your beautiful body, which has the power to give life, is more than worthy of that respect.

FINDING YOURSELF IN THE HARDEST OF PLACES

Sometimes it is a crisis that drives us to realize the urgent need to care for ourselves. Courtney sought therapy when his father killed himself. And years later, he reached for and held on to the Bible when he found himself teetering on the edge of a nervous breakdown.

His journey is a reminder that no experience is wasted. No one welcomes pain, but it is often the most difficult episodes that impart the most wisdom, including the discovery of what soothes our mind and soul. You can learn those lessons even in the harshest of places, under the most trying of circumstances, like when you are behind bars.

To be locked up is devastating. Dealing with the literal oppression of bars and guards can fuel depression and anxiety. Jail can also be the manifestation of a life-long fear that so many Black men have.

Even when you're out in the world, you often may not feel you have control over your life. Perhaps you feel, and rightly so, that the cards are stacked against you. My colleague Howard Stevenson and I often talk about how Black people in general feel damned if they do, damned if they don't, and just plain damned. We study hard, go on to college, and are still typically paid less than our white peers. We treat others with kindness, obey the rules, and still they may be pulled over, harassed, or even killed simply because a cop is having a bad day, or we were driving through the "wrong" neighborhood. We also know that an often corrupt, biased criminal justice system has laid traps to snare us all along the way.

So, for those who do actually wind up behind bars, whether their actions justify them being there or not, that confinement is often just a more visceral manifestation of what they experienced on the outside. Incarcerated people may have been able to walk around their home or their community. They may have had a steady job or even a big corporate title, but they were still scrutinized, demeaned, or judged. Their access and opportunity were still circumscribed by others. And now, with the little freedom and agency they had stripped away, their lifelong nightmare that they would end up where they are has finally come true.

Life behind bars also mirrors life on the outside in that it requires the wearing of a mask. Having a game face is one of the skill sets needed to survive in the larger world so you can keep that job or appear stoic or unafraid when a cop harasses you or a brother on the corner steps to you aggressively. And that mask continues to serve a vital purpose if you are locked within the violent, often sadistic world that is this nation's prison system. You hide your humanity so that you're left alone and can live long enough to one day make it out.

But while it can be a way to cope, constantly wearing a mask may also be a key reason so many young Black men get locked up in the first place, because ignoring your vulnerability only works for so long before you crumble or explode. Getting in touch with who you truly are can hopefully keep you from taking an action that robs you of your freedom. However, if you do tragically get caught up in this country's prison system, I've spoken to many men who say they've finally connected with their tenderness, their fears, and their internal questions while behind bars. With nothing but time, they became reflective, and began to search for the language to talk about dreams they didn't dare discuss when they were on the outside, trying to survive from day to day.

In his classic autobiography, written with Alex Haley, Malcolm X talked about reading the entire dictionary while he was incarcerated, honing his mind and eventually finding his spiritual mentor. Many other Black men who've spent time in prison recount how they got their high school diplomas or college degrees while there. Or perhaps they simply began to read about subjects they'd never thought much about for the very first time. They began to tap into their creativity, to pore through their imaginations. In this most terrible of settings, they learned how to tend to their selves.

Many also say that being behind bars drew them closer to their children. Some may have previously chosen not to be around their sons and daughters as much as they could. Others may have been blocked from seeing their children by ex-partners, or other circumstances. Being locked up made them appreciate their parental role all the more, and they wanted to do whatever they could to foster that irreplaceable relationship. They began to write to their children, constantly, and call them every chance they got.

They were becoming aware, to quote Bryan Stevenson, that they were so much more than the worst thing that they had done. Yes, they may have hurt someone, but at some point, they, too, were likely hurt. By reaching out to their children, they were taking the steps to end the cycle.

CARING FOR SELF TO CARE FOR EACH OTHER

I've met parents, partners, and older children who've begun their own internal work after their loved one goes to jail. They realize that if they want their father, husband, or son to be free one day and healthy, they need to look at themselves. After all, it's highly unlikely he got to the point where he committed an act that led to his imprisonment without dropping hints along the way that he was hurt or struggling. And so, by looking at their own behavior and experiences, family members can begin to heal their loved one and themselves too.

Perhaps they ask if their son erupted constantly with rage, was that something he learned growing up in a family that brawled at every holiday dinner and reunion? Or did he act up and act out because Dad didn't tolerate tears and Mom attributed every challenge or trauma to God's will?

There is power when a parent or a partner can own their own volatility, fears, or insecurities and talk about them with their injured loved one. There is power in saying, "I'm sorry I didn't know how to do this child-rearing, this loving, this partnering differently, but let's work on it together now, so you will be healthier emotionally wherever you are." Their introspection can be helped along by counseling, by meditating, or whatever activity helps them find a quiet place inside that allows them to contemplate and grow.

So many Black men end up meeting their humanity in a place set up to dehumanize them. I want to invite all Black men to examine the limitations that have been put on them by others, expectations that they may mistakenly call their own. Because when they internalize the lie that they are all swagger and no substance, sex machines and not tender beings, they lock themselves in a prison whether or not they ever set foot behind actual bars.

A LINE IN THE SAND

Self-care also means drawing boundaries.

Don't feel pressured to always take part in an activity with a romantic partner or even a friend. Maybe you want to go hear music, learn a new skill, or visit a museum by yourself. You may need something that feeds and fuels you and you, alone. Period. Full stop. There's no need to apologize or explain.

Consciously think about your boundaries, what works for you and what doesn't, when it comes to your interactions with others as well. That's not just self-care. That's self-respect. If there is someone who is exhausting you physically or mentally, with their criticism, their scrutiny, their raging, that is someone you may need to eliminate from your life. Or you may need to have a conversation with them, to let them know what you will tolerate and what you won't.

That goes for those who are the closest to you. Even perhaps the beloved woman who raised you.

The relationship between a mother and son is incredibly special. And given that many Black women have raised their sons on their own, the loyalty between them can be even more immense. But such bonds are also nuanced, and like any relationship, there may be moments of misunderstanding or discord. Some of those episodes may leave a lasting emotional imprint, yet it may be hard for a man to tell his mother how there were times he didn't get from her what he needed, or times still when the way she behaves leaves him feeling upset, disrespected, or unheard.

That's not a criticism. Black mothers have much to bear. They are raising Black boys in a hostile world. Often they are working outside the home as well as within it. And still so many do an amazing job, providing everything their children materially need, while filling them with encouragement and love.

But all that may not always be enough. Perhaps, as she juggled so many responsibilities and obligations, she didn't make room to listen to her son when he simply wanted to say he missed his mommy when she was out working all day—and that haunts him still. Or maybe, now that he's grown, she refuses to recognize that her constant interjecting, squabbling, or complaining is wearing him out.

And so her son may have to talk to her about what he was missing as he grew up. Or if her behavior in the here and now is often negative, even toxic, he must draw a boundary, the same line he is perhaps able to etch with his significant other, or a friend, but has struggled to establish with the woman who raised him.

I understand that's not easy to do. It's also hard to know what boundaries you need without doing some work, asking yourself the questions we've previously talked about—Who am I? Where does it hurt? It's only then that you can truly figure out what causes you distress.

"When you ask me a question and I try to answer, you cut me off. And that leaves me feeling frustrated."

"Whenever I tell you about an ambition I have, you put it down, and that discourages me."

Telling the person how their words stir, discourage or frustrate you, is a step forward, but that's not enough. You need to then tell them you are drawing a line in the sand. "When you cut me off, I get frustrated. So, when you do it, I'm going to end the call." Or, "We'll pick up the conversation when you're ready to listen. But in the meantime, I'm leaving the room." That's setting a boundary.

We often cling to the fantasy that our loved ones will see how upset we get when they pick arguments, offer excessive criticism, or refuse to listen, and so we won't have to set a marker because they change their behavior on their own.

"My father will stop hassling me."

"My partner will get that I'm tired right now and understand that I will eventually get to what they want me to do."

But change rarely happens without you having to do the work. A boundary is a clear definable action that keeps you safe and honors your feelings and experience—and you have to set it. It's not that you don't care about that other person's feelings. It's just that your feelings can't take a back seat to theirs. And once you establish what you will or won't tolerate, even if that other person in your life is miffed at first, chances are they'll eventually realize you did what was right and healthy for you. Boundaries can be a life saver and a life giver.

As you work toward becoming the whole, healthy being you are entitled to be, you must also embrace the power to create relationships that work for you. By establishing parameters that bring in what gives you nourishment and blocks out what depletes you, you are taking a stand, declaring to yourself and the world that you have immeasurable value, and you are worthy of protection.

SEEK AND DON'T HIDE

Black boys and men are also worthy of play, of experiencing unmitigated, unrelenting Black joy.

You deserve to revel in pleasure and frivolity. That means being able to be childlike even if you're grown. That means being comfortable engaging in an activity that society might typically define as "soft" or that some of your peers reject as "something other folks do, but not us."

No one can dictate how something makes you feel, and so there's no need to hide or deny whatever revives your spirit.

Not long ago, "Black men frolicking" was trending on social media. The videos showed brothers running and even skipping through fields. Some lay down on the grass. They were smiling, laughing, and clearly feeling elated.

Feel free to frolic. Walk barefoot through a mud patch if it makes you happy. Plant a garden. Pick up a hula hoop. Plunge into a pool.

It's important that Black men, abused and exploited for so long, be encouraged to explore what brings them pleasure both with, and apart from, their families and partners. For Black men and boys, who are so often attacked and disparaged, honoring yourselves is the greatest gift you can receive, because not only does it safeguard your physical and emotional health, but those acts of self-care can give you the energy you need to support all those who are in your concentric circles of friendship and love.

And it's essential that you think about what outside forces you let in that can shatter your sense of peace. Tune out the social media from time to time. If watching those constant reels of Black men being hurt becomes too debilitating—and how could it not?—don't watch. You've seen what happens. You've seen more than enough.

That selectivity can apply to the art you absorb as well. A rap may have a great beat, but does it spike your adrenaline or make you feel nervous? That song might be just what you need to take that extra lap around the track, but is it what you need to hear when you're about to have a conversation with your partner, or when you're trying to unwind after a hard day at work?

It's all connected. We're all connected. Your mental health affects your physical body. It impacts how well you can support your partner, your children, your parents. And wellness can also be infectious, inspiring others to make it a priority, rippling through a family or a neighborhood, helping an entire community to heal. Joy can be contagious. So take good care.

WHAT TO TAKE AWAY

✳ **Self-care is essential.** You can't support others if your well is dry and your tank is on empty.

✳ **Remember, your body is sacred.** Your body is a sacred vessel. Just as no one has the right to abuse you, don't abuse yourself. Sex for the sake of having sex is not necessarily healthy or gratifying. Consider your partners and protect your physical health.

✳ **Draw a line in the sand.** You are worthy of boundaries. Define what you will and will not tolerate.

✳ **Play.** Don't worry about how it appears to someone else. If it's not hurting you or others in your life, revel in what gives you respite and joy.

CHAPTER 10

On Community

"There is always light, if only we're brave enough to see it. If only we're brave enough to be it."

—AMANDA GORMAN

The Cort Theatre is like so many of those glorious vaudeville-era palaces dotting Broadway. There are gilded balconies and rows of tight seats. The narrow halls and cramped dressing rooms smell of perfume and dust and sweat.

Near the end of the summer of 2022, I visited the Cort for an amazing moment. I was there to celebrate a christening. The Cort was being renamed the James Earl Jones Theatre.

I remember how the sidewalk overflowed with celebrities and dignitaries. New York City's new mayor, Eric Adams, was there, and he said a few words. Journalists jostled each other with their notebooks and cameras. I walked the step and repeat, stopping to talk to various reporters. I'd done four or five short interviews when another gentleman approached. He asked a question I'd already answered several times. How did it feel to be here as this legendary theater was being renamed for James Earl Jones?

I started to speak, but the words caught in my throat. I tried again but I still couldn't utter a sound. Finally, I became overcome with emotion, I broke down, and my tears flowed. I tried to regain my composure, but I couldn't. I mumbled an apology to the reporter and quickly walked away.

What came over me in that moment was the overwhelming awe I felt realizing I knew the great James Earl Jones, and he knew me. Me. Courtney B. Vance, who grew up on Appoline Street. Me, a student athlete raised in Detroit, who had to learn what the word "upstaging" meant and so much more. Me, the young man who took a chance on acting simply to fulfill a promise I'd made to a high school teacher.

It hit me like a hammer from on high that here I was invited to praise the man who had been Troy Maxson, and that I'd had the privilege to play his son. Look at God, I thought. I made so many decisions by flipping a coin in my head, but God was always there, placing the people I didn't know I needed in my path, weaving the circle of friends and griots who enabled me to be who and where I am.

What came over me was appreciation. What came over me was gratitude. All that divine guidance and all those blessings were encapsulated in that moment in Midtown Manhattan, and it just blew me away.

We all need a tribe, those folks who glimpse the potential in us that we can't see in ourselves. Those people who pull us into an embrace when they know we are hurting or point us in the right direction when we have lost our way.

My family and neighborhood in Detroit gave me a foundation. The Boys' Club gave me a nurturing place to grow and play. A teacher at Country Day gave me a role and a suggestion that paved the way to my professional destiny.

But not everyone is so fortunate. I know that I have many

Black brothers who struggle to find community. That's why each of us has to look out for the boy who is sullen or shy, the man who may be hiding his pain behind bluster or a bottle, and the guy at the office who is quick to anger. Black men need those ties that bind more than most because of the extraordinary pressures we endure being who we are in an often-hostile world. We need that safety net to catch us. We need that village to affirm what we have to offer, reassure us that our frustrations are justified, and to give us a safe place to unburden our minds. Community can help save our lives.

Like many teenagers, I didn't have a clear idea what career I wanted to get into. Because I'd heard somewhere in my childhood that my father wanted to be an attorney, I had a faint interest in the law, and I did an internship during my senior year of high school at a law firm. But I wasn't feeling all those arcane statutes and terms. Then, I briefly thought architecture might be interesting, so I took a mechanical drawing class. But it scared me to think that if I was off by a sixteenth of an inch, those big walls I designed could come tumbling down.

So, when I was accepted to Harvard, I decided to be a history major simply because that was a subject I loved. I figured I could settle on what I wanted to do professionally after I'd spent some time exploring different subjects, in class and around campus.

In the meantime, I decided to participate in Country Day's senior play. Ronnie Clemmer, the show's director, was also an assistant football coach I'd gotten to know during my years on the team. And like pretty much everyone else at school, I really loved him. Mr. Clemmer also taught English, and he was that cool young teacher who introduced countless young minds to the magic of *Beowulf, The Canterbury Tales*, and so many other literary classics. I was in honors English and so I never got to take his class, but I was able to spend some time under Mr. Clemmer's tutelage when I got a part in the senior production.

I don't think I had more than three lines, but I had a whole lot of fun, and Mr. Clemmer encouraged me to stick with it.

"You've got talent, Courtney," he said. "Promise me you'll continue acting when you get to Harvard."

I smiled, told him I would, and pushed his suggestion to the back of my mind.

When I did get to Harvard, I went back to what I knew to anchor myself—sports—and I was eager to get back with the guys and run track. I was raring to go, working out before class in the morning, doing sprints on my own in the afternoon. I went to the coach's office one day in early fall to find out the practice schedule.

"Courtney," he said, looking up from some papers he'd been riffling through. "We don't run until December. Go study."

Track season couldn't come soon enough. I always loved being part of a team, setting a collective goal that a group of us could work to reach together. But to my surprise, after just a few practices, I felt bored.

This ain't fun, I thought. I've been here, done this. I wanted to meet new people with different interests. And that was especially important to me because I was still trying to figure out what I wanted to pursue professionally.

I'd visited the career services office, but they had nothing but a bunch of business cards with outdated phone numbers. Then one day, I happened to strike up a conversation with a student who was part of the campus's theater scene. I suddenly remembered what I'd told Mr. Clemmer.

I'd already earned a varsity letter as a second hurdler on the track team. I played three sports all through high school. What more did I have to prove? I decided to make a change. After the last race of the season, when I'd cleared my final hurdle, I went to Coach Frank Haggarty and told him I was quitting the team.

He was very disappointed, but he understood and wished me the best.

I had a whole plan for where my theater adventure would lead. I envisioned meeting new people with every production and my fellow actors would talk to me about what their parents did for a living and their own ambitions. That's what I was looking for—new connections and new perspectives. Acting was a means to that end.

It didn't disappoint. The theater crowd was tight knit and dynamic. We'd improvise scenes and riff late into the night. We became like family, and I was doubly fortunate because I had two villages, my theater crew and Harvard's community of Black students.

It was different than Country Day, where the handful of Black kids floated through, not avoiding each other but not really bonding either. At Harvard, we hung tight. We had plenty of classes where we were the only one, or one of the very few like us, in the room. But once class ended, we were together, discussing politics in Harvard Yard, attending concerts by the Black choir Kuumba, or partying to Michael Jackson and Chaka Khan in one of the Houses, our name for the dorms.

We'd sometimes get curious looks from our white peers. I've always found it hilarious when a white person wonders why Black folks always seem to hang around each other. My response includes a few questions: "Why do *y'all* always hang with each other? Do you invite us in? Do you want to hang around with us? If you do, come on. If you don't, be quiet."

I'll say again that I have friends and mentors from all backgrounds. Like Mr. George Browne at the Boys' Club, who shepherded all of us kids and recommended Country Day to my family. Like Mr. Robert Stone, head of worldwide purchasing at GM, who took me under his wing with an amazing summer job and an introduction to his boss, Mr. Charles Fuller, who promised to put me through Harvard Business School when I was a rising junior at Harvard.

I also had many white teachers and coaches who inspired and encouraged me, including Mr. Ronnie Clemmer, who's now a producer in Los Angeles and is a friend of mine to this day, and Mrs. Beverly Hannett-Price, my Country Day Honors English teacher, who is still teaching after sixty-five years.

But sometimes, as a Black person—as a Black man—you need to be surrounded by people who mirror you. You need to be with folks who understand the cultural cues and codes, the slights and swipes without you having to codeswitch, or explain a thing. You need the person who speaks your language without your having to translate, and who can help create a space where you can vent without apology and simply celebrate being you.

———

Just as a good word from a beloved teacher got me on the path to acting, community looked out for me when I took a step that almost cost me everything.

When I decided to try out for the Yale School of Drama and was accepted, I was making a commitment to acting. But I was surrounded by some of the most gifted raw talents in the country and so there was no guarantee that Lloyd Richards, the first African American Dean, would pick me out of the crowd. Yet he did, casting me as Cory in *Fences*.

Like all of August Wilson's plays that debuted at Yale, the productions went on the road, where they could be tested before audiences far beyond New Haven. Yale frowned on students doing professional work and so I shouldn't have been allowed to play Cory off campus. But though I was a third-year student, Lloyd brought me to Chicago with the rest of the cast. That was the first no-no, initiated by Lloyd, who was literally running the show. The next one would be all on me.

Hollywood was casting a film based on Richard Wright's classic novel *Native Son*, and the producers had been looking for the actor who would play the protagonist, Bigger Thomas, for a year. Don't ask me how I heard about a casting call taking place in Chicago, or what I was thinking when I decided to go check it out. Maybe one of the other actors in *Fences* mentioned it, or I read about it in the *Chicago Tribune* or a trade paper while riding the El train. Anyway, I did my usual mental coin flip one afternoon when I was free and decided to stop by the theater where they were holding auditions.

They asked me to read. And boom. I was Bigger Thomas.

I had a chance to costar in a major motion picture with Matt Dillon, Elizabeth McGovern, and Oprah Winfrey, the shot of a lifetime. But Yale had strict rules. The school was so close to New York City, if it allowed students to pursue professional roles, none of us would ever finish our degree. And I knew in a couple months, my classmates and I were supposed to head to the culmination of all of our work at the Yale School of Drama—The League Auditions— held at Juilliard every year, where we'd perform monologues and scenes with the hope of being signed by one of the agents in attendance. I turned the role down and let Lloyd know. We planned to see each other back on campus the following Tuesday.

But the film's producers weren't ready to give up. They began calling Yale alumni, telling them that Lloyd was pressuring me to not accept the role, which wasn't true. Before the final performance of *Fences* that Sunday night, Lloyd and I spoke again and unfortunately we totally misunderstood each other. He now thought I wanted to take the part of Bigger, and I thought he was telling me that I should. So now I was confused. We'd been in agreement in our first conversation but now I didn't know what he was telling me to do. I was at a crossroads and would have to decide for myself.

I knew I had to get back with my class and finish school. Members of the *Native Son* cast were going to do a table read that Monday. Oprah, Matt, Elizabeth. And me.

I asked Frankie Faison, who was playing the part of Gabe in *Fences,* what he thought I should do.

"Court, I don't know what to tell you," Frankie said, looking at me with more pity than excitement. "It's Bigger Thomas. That's a great role."

"I know," I responded. "But. But. I'm in school."

Frankie told me he knew it was a really tough call, and he was there to listen, but he couldn't make the decision for me. I was up until 4:00 in the morning, twisting in the sheets, weighing the pros and cons until my head hurt. Exhausted, I did the reading. Then later that day, I grabbed my suitcases and headed back to Yale.

I went to see the Yale School of Drama's associate dean, Earl Gister, to tell him what happened and ask him how I could handle the situation. We had a very good relationship.

"Court," he said. "You're out."

The room began to spin.

"You did the reading," he continued. "You're not supposed to do professional work while you're a student here. You knew that. So you're out."

I was in shock and started asking if there was anything I could do. He asked if I had signed any papers, and when I told him I hadn't, he said to call the producers and tell them I couldn't take the part.

"Earl," I said, "since I don't have an agent, you make the call as my representative." He did, and all hell broke loose.

Once again, folks didn't say what I needed to hear.

"What do you mean, you aren't going to do it?" the producers screamed when I took the receiver. "We've been looking for Bigger for a year, and you're it! You auditioned. You did a reading. You're going to do this!"

The phone in the apartment I shared with my girlfriend, the phone in Mr. Gister's office, and the phone at my parents' home rang off the hook for the next three days. The producers called me so much, my girlfriend and I fled to New York to get away from it. My mother took to her bed, worried sick. The producers threatened to sue. It was a nightmare.

In addition to being worried, my parents were mystified. "We thought you wanted to do this, Son," they said. "Isn't the whole point of going to drama school to get a big part in a movie?"

Looking back now, I realize that crisis was not just a pivotal moment in my professional journey; it represented a point between my usual impulsive decision making and the maturity that years later would enable me to be still while I waited for my thoughts to clear.

I was at a crossroads. I had the support of my family, who would back me no matter what. I also had my girlfriend's love, and the sympathetic ear of friends like Frankie Faison. Their presence gave me the strength to make a decision that had to be my own.

I'd made a commitment to my classmates and myself when I enrolled at Yale. I wasn't supposed to do professional work while I was there. Lloyd had violated that rule by allowing me to go to Chicago. I would be forever grateful for the trust he had in me and the heat he took, but I knew I couldn't do *Native Son*. I had to finish school and let this golden opportunity go. There would be others.

My classmates were still furious, and probably more than a little jealous. The first time we all met after I'd turned down the part, our amazing voice teacher, Ms. Zoe Alexander, let everyone say what they were feeling, yelling at me for at least an hour before my girlfriend, forever in my corner, said that was enough and quieted everyone down. We finally got back to getting ready for our League Auditions. The calls from the film's producers also eventually stopped, and they went on to cast the wonderful actor Victor Love as Bigger instead.

I didn't feel any particular joy when *Native Son* was released a year or two later and tanked at the box office. It was an important story in the American literary canon, with a stellar cast, including Love, who became a good friend.

But after I went to Juilliard with the rest of my class and got my Hollywood agent. After I saw the reviews for the film I'd turned down. After I went on to do *Fences* on Broadway, it was more than clear that I'd done the right thing.

Not everybody is worthy to be in your community. You have to be discerning. There are people who just want to criticize, and not because they're being constructive but because they want to tear you down. I've had a few people I had to leave along the way when our so-called friendships were no longer healthy for me. And sometimes you have to test folks. You let them in a little, telling them about a triumph you've had or a problem you're pondering, and then you sit back, watch, and listen. Do they interrupt and make the conversation all about them? Do they resent your happiness or enjoy your insecurity? Or are they willing to bask in your achievement, or maybe just quietly listen as you unload?

I remember hearing that Dr. Martin Luther King Jr. would hold three- or four-hour meetings, letting all his lieutenants scream and argue while he didn't say a word. Then, when they were hoarse and worn out, he'd stand up, synthesize all their speechifying into a two-minute sound bite, and decide what he and they were going to do. He was listening and he was watching to determine who was the right person to walk beside him. He was testing the waters to see on whom he could rely, who had something meaningful to say, and who was just out for themselves and not the cause.

Steve Jobs, the cofounder of Apple, did something similar. From what I understand, he'd write several items on a white board, leaving his team to narrow the list down to three, and then he'd come back to them after a couple of days and change it up, saying actually there was only one point that mattered. The people who could hang during that whittling process were the people he knew he could go to war with, like Gideon in the Bible, who goes to the river with 10,000 men, but sets out for battle with just 300.

I'm not saying that friendship or love should be a hazing, that people have to fight a death match to prove they deserve to be in your life. What I am saying is that we all need someone that we can lean on when we're having trouble standing on our own. Maybe they falter too, because they are going through their own struggles, and after all, we are all only human. Maybe you have to be the shoulder that holds firm for them and put your own troubles on hold because friendship has to be a give-and-take.

But ultimately, after enough time and situations, it becomes clear who is in our corner for the bad times as well as the good. And if someone takes and never shares, if they always have something negative to say and nothing positive to give, you might want to consign them to a small part of your life—if they remain in your world at all.

There are also folks who are in your life for a season, and no more. I continued to care about my old buddies on Appoline Street, but our journeys eventually had little in common. Beyond our memories, which held a special place, we just didn't have much more to share.

And then there are those you don't stay in constant touch with, but whose support and wisdom you'll always treasure and never forget.

Years after I'd finished my work with Dr. K, I reached out to her again. I was getting married to Angela and I wanted Dr. K at our wedding.

"Courtney," Dr. K said after the ceremony. "We did some good work."

"We did?" I said. I'd had no idea that she felt me getting my dreams the way I did was some of the most rewarding work of her professional life. There was no editing with us. Through my dreams, Dr. K was able to see exactly how to help me quickly.

Look at God, I thought, how he orchestrated my life so I could keep going and growing. Leslie and Conroy. Grunilla and Dr. K. James and Mary Alice.

The Great Conductor had convened a community for me. Time and again my community saved me. And it continues to give me the sustenance and the humility I need to be a connector, to do all that I can to help lift up all my brothers, letting them know that we can stumble through the darkness together and collectively summon the spark that helps us all to carry on.

A New Movement, a New Momentum

Black people, forced to come to what some proclaimed a "new world," were from diverse places on a faraway continent. They spoke different languages and had different traditions. But once they were thrown together, strangers in a brutal land, they clung to each other. And we have held each other ever since.

In many ways, Black people have defined the culture of this nation, providing its artistic heartbeat while being its conscience, pushing it to make its hollow promises whole. And our solidarity is now sparking a new movement, one that is creating and cultivating the language, spaces, and resources that will empower Black boys and men to speak their truths out loud and become the fully realized human beings they were born to be.

Yes, we continue to live in a racist, sexist society, capable of horrific acts of violence against our bodies and psyches. But Black people are not waiting idly for systems created to burden and break us to tell our stories in Hollywood, to bring an end to state violence, or to invest in our communities. We're doing this for ourselves.

And just as Black people are taking artistic and economic initiative on our own behalf, we are also taking steps collectively to ensure our mental wellness.

Those efforts range from the Just Heal, Bro Tour, which invites men to gather and mirror one another with the guidance of trained professionals, to the support group for grieving Black fathers created by Bruce McIntyre III and Omari Maynard. There are therapists and community advocates making a point to offer counseling, sometimes at no cost, to Black boys and men who seek it. And there are Black men in the spotlight who are using their platforms to speak about the importance of their brothers preserving and strengthening their emotional health.

A movement is happening because momentum is building. There is an ever-growing recognition among Black people, and Black men in particular, that they deserve more. And they are also realizing as they raise a new generation that they can change the paradigm, making mental health as much of a priority as going to school, paying bills, or attending church was for previous generations.

It's not that we don't appreciate the power of faith that has held Black people in good stead during the most hellish of times. Courtney, like so many others, prays and keeps his Bible at the ready. But Black people as a whole are also waking up to the reality that coping with stress, healing from emotional injury, and reaching for joy require many tools and new ways of thinking.

Therapy is one. A new model for masculinity is another. You may need to take medication, or to write regularly in a journal so when it's difficult to open up to an outsider, you can at least be vulnerable with yourself. And as a people, we are realizing that to have widespread emotional healing, we need a collective commitment.

MAKING AN INTENTIONAL CONNECTION

Creating and maintaining community requires being proactive. Banding together was easier decades ago. Extended families often lived within blocks or a few miles of each other. Grandparents, aunts, and uncles may have all lived in the same household. But today, that's rarely the case. As a result, many young Black men and boys haven't experienced the same feeling of connection that buoyed their grandparents and ancestors. Nowadays, we have to connect with intention.

When the coach reaches out to the boy on the pee wee football team, when the neighbor speaks to the teenager who rakes his leaves come October, when the commuter speaks to the kid at the bus station who may have no home at all, it may be the first time someone has asked that young person how they are doing and really wanted to hear their heartfelt answer.

Mental health professionals can also train coaches, principals, and businesspeople on how to guide tender conversations. Then Black men can reach out to each other in the moment—right after the foul ball or the misguided slight, right before a punch is thrown or a spark is lit. They can be equipped with the phone numbers or social media handles of those who can build on the support they immediately give, because treatment doesn't have to be on a couch or in a therapist's office. Counseling can happen right where Black boys and men are—in a barber's chair, on a basketball court, or in a community center gym.

Just as a barber can become more conscious of the therapeutic role he or she plays, all of us can do more to bolster the Black boys and men in our lives. Healing can come from a beloved elder who listens with empathy, or a good friend who asks questions with compassion. We can gently prod our neighbors, students, or loved ones to speak honestly about how they feel, and we can match the stories they tell with our own. When we empower each other, change happens, and it clears the path for an ever-growing number of Black men and boys to find peace.

FINDING A ROCK TO STAND ON

There is also something that every Black man can do on his own, for free. You can purposefully seek out people whom you trust and who trust you. You can create a small support group of your own. Like that beautiful group of young men who were close to my nephew Kenney. Like the professionals who came together in that gathering I counseled in a Denver hotel ballroom several years ago.

Of course, there must be ground rules. People must commit to confidentiality and honor. But that needs to be established in any environment, whether it's the office of a professional therapist, or a church's prayer circle. There's always a need for people to make sure they feel protected, that they can be vulnerable without fear or judgment. But once you have vetted those with whom you want to share, you have an invaluable touchstone you can turn to whenever you are in need.

None of this is to say that the mental health of Black men and boys shouldn't be of concern to the broader society. This country has long thrived from the literal labor and cultural contributions of Black men and boys, a group that, despite terrible discrimination, fought valiantly in every war, operated the machinery of industry from Detroit to Oakland, and sketched the American story with their lyrics, painting, and prose. The government that enshrined redlining and segregation, the courts that continue to mete out injustice, and the schools that stigmatize and undereducate, all have a role to play in eliminating the inequities that too often leave Black boys and men fragile, frustrated, and frightened.

But Black men, on their own, are lifting the silence that has shrouded their hurt for too long. By stripping away the masks you often wear in public, you are enabling others to bare their true selves and give voice to their experiences. You are upending the lie that expressing pain makes you weak, spreading the good news that you can be both resilient and fragile, vulnerable and strong. You are letting your sons and fathers know that they have the right to speak, that they have the right to cry out, and that they have an obligation to themselves and their maker to explore what makes them deep down happy.

SHOULD YOU FORGIVE AND FORGET?

Of course, people are complicated. The wounds we accumulate in life inevitably come from interactions we have. A lover may let you down. A sibling may be difficult and distant. A friend may betray you or disappear in your hour of need.

And so, to be healthy mentally, should you forgive them?

Forgiveness is important but not in the way that many people think. Often when we talk about forgiving, we think about it in the context of granting grace to others. But it's most important to grant grace to ourselves. That means getting to the point where you can look at the holes you carry inside and accept their presence no matter who put them there.

Or maybe it was you who treated an old friend or partner in a way you now regret. Perhaps you were raised by a parent who told you that you couldn't trust anybody, and so you are blaming yourself for the suspicion you've carried for all these years that kept you from letting in love and affection. Maybe you were unfaithful in a relationship or mean-spirited to someone who'd always treated you with kindness.

It's critical that we look at the roots of our actions, the events and episodes and people who helped shape us. But as you search for that understanding, extend an olive branch to yourself. Always remember that you are so much more than your faults. You are greater than all the negative things that were done to you. Your weaknesses create opportunities for you to reflect and evolve. Your trials enable you to feel compassion for others. No circumstance is without meaning. No experience is wasted. They are all fragments that, when stitched together, make us who we are, ragged edges and all.

Forgiveness doesn't mean excusing the hurtful actions of others. It's not giving up your power and opening the door to be retraumatized or abused. You don't have to make peace with a partner who beat you, or grab coffee with the one-time friend who told your secrets. You don't have to reengage with the person or the system that harmed you. If anything, it is healthier, if at all possible, to stay far away.

But as you think about forgiveness, once again, language is important. We need new words to reframe our thinking. Maybe instead of forgiveness, we talk about understanding. Instead of forgiveness, we talk about acceptance. Because if you understand how not getting your needs met by your parents left you impatient with your spouse, how an unstable youth fueled your depression, or how discrimination at a job left you anxious and lacking in confidence, you can start taking steps to quiet those voices while also accepting that you can't go back in time to change the past.

It doesn't mean you're okay with whoever might have hurt you. But you can begin to understand how their behavior impacted you, then move forward. You can gain clarity about why you feel the way you feel and why you react the way you react. You are solving riddles, resolving questions, and that allows you to make room to accept who you are, fully.

Develop a mantra to guide your inner work. "I know this happened. It was wrong. It hurt. I can't change it. But I can also grant myself a fresh beginning. I am worthy of all goodness and grace."

Write those words down. Run them through your mind. Say them out loud if you can. Then turn your gaze toward the future.

Acceptance and understanding are a part of self-care. They are integral to being able to open up, connect with others, and create community. And like all aspects of healing, they are actions you have to commit to practicing until your heart takes its last beat.

I often meet people who say they have overcome something. That they've been delivered. I'm glad they feel peace in the moment, but I have to break it to them that their tranquility may not be everlasting.

They may feel unsettled again tomorrow, the next day, or next week. To fully accept and move past layers of trauma is a constant exercise. Your goal to keep pain in the rearview mirror has to be set anew every day. Being at ease with pieces of your past can come and go. But the point is to keep trying, keep moving toward your highest good.

Seek out the spaces where you can excavate your emotions. Look for the folks who will ask you questions and help you find solutions. Lean on the friend or mentor who can help you ferret out what's working for you, what isn't, and what other resources are out there to help you make a meaningful change.

DOING THE WORK THAT'S WORTH IT

Barber shops and boys' and girls' clubs. Fraternities and recreation centers. Social media. Television and hip hop.

The village comes in many forms, and there are so many within it who can catch you when you stumble.

Efforts like the National Mental Health Initiative have the potential to broadly do a lot of good for everyone. But there remains a need to specifically reach out to Black boys and men in a way that's focused and authentic. And the more the Black community talks about the need to tend to our collective mental health, and spotlights all the ways how, the more wellness can become the norm and not a rarity.

We are steadily making Black men's mental wellness part of the everyday. That's what happens when there's an episode of *Atlanta* that lifts up therapy, when a DJ puts on the Geto Boys' "Mind Playing Tricks on Me" in the middle of an old-school mix, or when Courtney takes the stage to talk about the forces that led to his father's and godson's suicides.

Social media, while imperfect, can also be a vital platform where those who are seeking and struggling can find community. Currently, TikTok is full of testimonies from young people detailing their experiences with sorrow, creating a port in the storm for all those who are suffering. And people like Kier Gaines, a therapist who recounts his journey navigating relationships, parenting, and other aspects of life as a Black man in America for his hundreds of thousands of followers, provide a mirror and a road map to all those walking similar paths.

So all of you trying to become your most fully realized selves should know that there are so many who are rooting for you. You should know that there are legions ready, willing, and waiting to mirror not only your struggles, but also your humanity and your divine potential.

Feeling comfortable exploring and expressing your emotions takes time and effort. It's just like exercising a muscle. Going to the gym a couple times a year won't do. It must be constant. It can be hard. But it is important. It may even be a matter of life and death. And there are so many others doing the same work who are willing to offer a helping hand.

For the broader community of Black people and their allies, the work can sometimes appear daunting, as crises and events continue to break your heart. Not so long ago, for instance, in Philadelphia, a fourteen-year-old boy was killed. He was a young football player, participating in a scrimmage at a school he didn't attend because his school didn't have a team. When the game was over, in the middle of the afternoon, a group of other Black teenagers showed up and began shooting. In the blink of an eye, a fourteen-year-old was dead, and several other teenagers had committed a crime that would likely send them to prison for the rest of their lives.

Stories like that, especially when it involves Black boys hurting each other, can make you wither. But while such tragedies need to be acknowledged, we can't ignore the many efforts taking place to prevent them from happening at all. Courtney and Jay Barnett, J. Ivy and Kenny Lattimore, Howard Stevenson and radio personality Charlamagne tha God, are among the many Black men who are taking their brothers by the shoulders and asking, How are you doing, truly? Where do you hurt? How can I help? They are pouring love and positivity into their brothers, acknowledging their challenges while also reflecting back to them their talents and beauty.

So, despite the scale of the task and the toll of the heartbreak, I am encouraged.

As you do your inner work, you may have to grab a gulp of air like you do before diving into the deep end of a pool.

You may have to make a personal determination each and every day to peer inside and take on the tasks that can keep you emotionally stable and well.

That wound you thought was healed may reopen. You might feel ready to move on from an old injury one day, only to find yourself welling up with fear or anger a few weeks later. But that's where community comes in. That is its divine purpose. Because healing is a process, and every day, every hour, may summon a new challenge, but community can provide the lifelines that help you make it through.

CREATING YOUR OWN

Amid all the work that it takes to make a living, nurture a family, and keep yourself healthy so you can be there for others as well as yourself, Black men must also never forget to make time to play, to discover and revel in whatever makes their soul sing. And when we create recreational spaces for our Black youth, let us always remember that every environment is a reflection of those within it, so let's give them a place that mirrors how special they are.

Let's make sure that hoop some of the kids congregate around has a net and not just a rickety rim. Put fresh paint on the walls of that community center. Bring in healthy snacks. Illuminate those young men's humanity by letting them know they're worthy of a space that is clean, safe, and inviting.

Here's what else all of us who love Black boys and men can do: We can encourage them to cry in public and not criticize or turn away from them when they do. We can remind them that they are glorious human beings who, no matter what they've endured, can still set goals and achieve.

Community can provide the protection that allows Black men and boys to Wake Up! Show Up! Grow Up! Rise Up!™ to seize their dreams and future. It can provide the space where they can be vulnerable and speak about their burdens and concerns. Community can create the places where Black men and boys can break free from the hypermasculine cast that stifles their emotions, the straitjacket that forces so many to move through life as a character or a stereotype, rather than as their authentic selves.

And then, when they are given that opening to fully be who they are, they can also become healthier fathers, partners, and sons. They are able to model for the next generation how to live fulfilled lives. And given how much Black men have been able to accomplish in the face of unthinkable odds, when they have the tools to come to grips with the emotional wounds we all must deal with, when they are no longer held hostage by their past and can redirect their energy into building and creating, they can accomplish the unimaginable.

Courtney and I have one final message for our brothers: Don't be afraid to ask the questions that can lead to the answers you are looking for.

Where does it hurt? What do I tell myself about me? Whose voice do I hear? Who is the real me?

By tending to their past hurts, Black men can tackle their present struggles. When they wake up to the experiences that may be holding them back, and take action to nurture themselves emotionally, they can rise up to become who they were meant to be.

That is nothing less than a holy endeavor. Health and wholeness are on the horizon. All you have to do is reach for them.

Acknowledgments

COURTNEY B. VANCE

It takes a village to nurture the publication of a book into being. We are blessed to have had the love, patience, and support of an amazing universe of people, from friends and family to those who have been, as well as have become, a treasured part of our lives as members of our respective teams.

We would like to thank our publishing home, Balance, our publisher Nana K. Twumasi, and Natalie Bautista, for keeping us on time, on track, and on purpose. We are grateful that you were aligned with us on the urgency and critical importance of this book and gave us the opportunity to offer *The Invisible Ache* to the world.

Charisse Jones, you are a true collaborator who has been instrumental in not only bringing together our voices but also giving each of us the space to offer our individual perspectives and experiences. You are a brilliant writer, but you're also a compassionate, soulful human being.

Our eternal thanks to friend and colleague Dr. Selena Sermeño, a psychologist deeply committed to promoting the human rights, healing, and empowerment of marginalized groups in the United States and abroad, and who lent her time and expertise to make sure we were aware of the most recent and pertinent research.

To literary agent Steve Troha, we deeply appreciate your paving the way for us to find a great home with Balance. And thank you to Simone Cooper and Gilda Squire for being our cheerleaders, champions, and publishing industry whisperers.

DR. ROBIN SMITH

This may be the most humbling part of writing a book—to acknowledge the great cloud of witnesses who leaned in to bring *The Invisible Ache* vibrantly alive. We thank our devastating pain and loss that called forth this creative work. We thank our fathers, our Daddies, Black men who faced layered complexity and gave us the best they had when so much was unjustly stolen and missing. And to our mothers, our Mommies, who held themselves and our families together, pointing the way to freedom that we might live more fully despite pain, isolation, and suffering.

I am because of my father and mother, now both on the other side and yet more with me than ever: Warren E. Smith, M.D., and Rosa Lee Smith, MSS; and to Damian and Joy, my twin brother and sister, and to a family who believes in my calling no matter the cost.

Without the invisible and yet purposeful hands and heart of God, we could have missed each other and this holy creative matrimony of coming together on this project and on others to follow. Gilda Squire, a GOAT for bringing us together. "Thank you" does not begin to capture the depth and breadth of appreciation we both feel for you, your keen vision, and your extraordinary giftedness in the entertainment and publishing worlds. Your partnership with Simone Cooper is a covering we honor, value, and cherish.

Our teams at Bassett Vance Productions and Fearless Won/

Dr. Robin are the epitome of ride, die, and live abundantly without exception, hesitation, or apology.

There is a tribe who walk and run with us, and hold us tenderly and accountable as we navigate our own Invisible Ache. A shout-out to the prolific work of friend, brother, and pioneer in the space of Black boys and men, as well as racial literacy, Dr. Howard C. Stevenson Jr.

REJ, the Black knight in human armor whose courageous heart and body befriend me as partner and friend. I honor your Invisible Ache, and your voice in the liberation of all people, especially Black men and boys.

Thank you to all the Black boys and men around the nation and world who shared their stories with us—as well as those who didn't live to tell their stories—and to the young and older brothers alike who somehow still rise and shine every day, who have game and are grand, free or behind bars. We see you, and *The Invisible Ache* is for you. Thank you for breathing and being...thank you!

About the Authors

Courtney B. Vance is an award-winning actor on stage, on film, and in television. His credits include historically noteworthy films such as *Hamburger Hill*, *The Hunt for Red October*, *The Preacher's Wife*, and *The Adventures of Huck Finn*. Courtney's portrayal of Johnnie Cochran in FX's *The People vs. OJ Simpson: American Crime Story*, of "Uncle George" in HBO's *Lovecraft Country*, and of Rev. C. L. Franklin in NatGeo's *Genius: Aretha* have earned him two Emmys, a Critics Choice Award, a Black Reel TV Award, and multiple NAACP Image Awards, as well as SAG, Golden Globe, and Hollywood Critics Association nominations. He won a Tony for his performance of Hap Hairston on Broadway in *Lucky Guy* and is the recipient of the Bounce Trumpet Award for Excellence in Entertainment and the ABFF Honors Award for Excellence in the Arts. Courtney earned a Grammy nomination for his narration of Neil DeGrasse Tyson's *Accessory to War*. His starring role on AMC Network's criminal justice drama *61st Street* earned him an African American Film Critics Association TV Honor. He is co-founder of Bassett Vance Productions with his wife, Angela Bassett. Courtney is also president of the SAG-AFTRA Foundation.

A #1 bestselling author, sought-after speaker, experienced media personality, ordained minister, and host of SiriusXM's

The Dr. Robin Show, **Dr. Robin L. Smith** addresses today's most pressing societal challenges through fearless truth-telling. As a licensed psychologist known for her signature four-step prescription Wake Up! Show Up! Grow Up! Rise Up!™, she brings a uniquely healing perspective to our nation's most daunting social justice and mental health issues: from systemic racism and racial violence, to grief and loss, to discrimination based on gender and sexual orientation, to recovering and rebounding as a nation following crises.

She was introduced to viewers globally during her years as the on-air therapist for *The Oprah Winfrey Show.* She currently works with major corporations, nonprofit organizations, and sports and entertainment professionals, leading breakthrough programs and presentations that help people overcome adversity.

Dr. Robin is the author of the *New York Times* #1 bestseller *Lies at the Altar: The Truth About Great Marriages,* which has been translated into 14 languages, as well as the soulful memoir *Hungry: The Truth About Being Full* and *Inspirational Vitamins: A Guide to Personal Empowerment.*

Dr. Robin has a PhD in counseling psychology from Temple University and a master's degree from Eastern Baptist Theological Seminary.